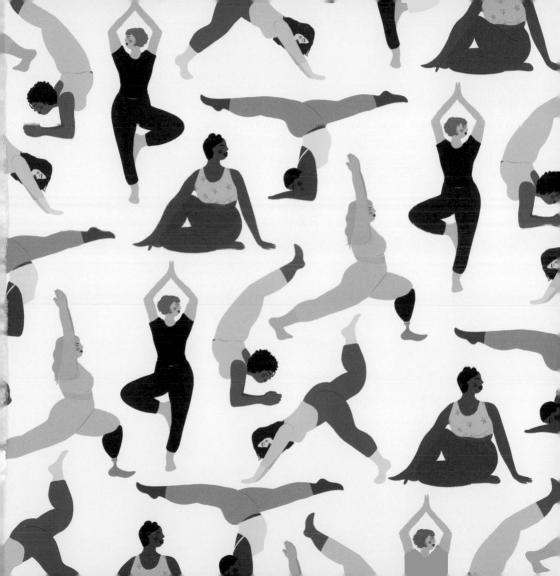

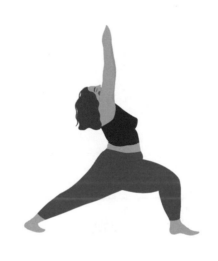

CELEBRATING THE YOGI IN ALL OF US

YOU ARE STRONG
STRONG
and
WORTHY

HARMONY WILLOW HANSEN

WORKMAN PUBLISHING • NEW YORK

Library of Congress Cataloging-in-Publication Data is available.

ISBN 978-1-5235-1440-3

Design by Lisa Hollander

Cover illustration by Harmony Willow Hansen

Workman books are available at special discounts when purchased in bulk for premiums and sales promotions as well as for fundraising or educational use. Special editions or book excerpts can also be created to specification. For details, please contact special.markets@hbgusa.com.

Workman Publishing Co., Inc.,
a subsidiary of Hachette Book Group, Inc.
1290 Avenue of the Americas
New York, NY 10104

workman.com

WORKMAN is a registered trademark of Workman Publishing Co., Inc.,
a subsidiary of Hachette Book Group, Inc.

Printed in China on responsibly sourced paper.

First printing February 2023

10 9 8 7 6 5 4 3 2 1

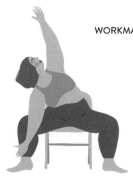

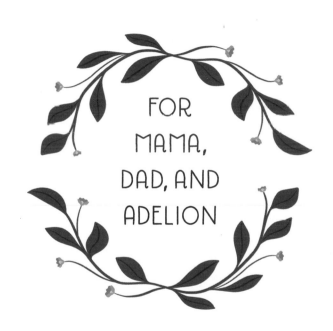

FOR
MAMA,
DAD, AND
ADELION

INTRODUCTION

I've practiced yoga for years. Early on I was scared and uncomfortable, always trying to find a spot in the back of the room so no one would notice me. That changed when I lived in LA and attended a yoga studio that employed twin red-headed actresses who were also in a rock band. They provided a space of joy and freedom for everyone, regardless of age or mobility. Most of the time, I was the youngest person by 40 years. Attending their classes made me really fall in love with yoga and realize that it wasn't about holding the pose for a long time or even being able to do every pose each time. Yoga was and is about connecting to yourself with kindness and giving yourself the freedom to rely solely on your own body. I think that's why I love yoga—because unlike so many workout routines, you need only your body. You could be anywhere in the world and go into warrior pose or close your eyes and practice your breathing. The beauty of yoga is that it's personal and yet millions of people are practicing all over the world, connecting us and bringing us closer to ourselves and those who share this joy. The word *yoga* comes from the Sanskrit word *Yuj*, which means "to join" or "to unite." Whether alone in our home or in a crowded yoga studio, we are uniting our bodies with our minds as well as uniting ourselves with everyone else practicing with us.

This book of illustrations was created to encourage, inspire, and spread unity throughout the yoga community—newcomers and experienced yogis alike. It's not intended to be a guide. It's a gathering of all kinds of yoga poses, showing every kind of body, with encouraging sayings sprinkled throughout. Many of the poses have both English and Sanskrit names. I created the names for several positions, therefore those do not have Sanskrit names.

I hope these illustrations fuel your practice, your joy, your dedication, and your appreciation for your amazing body.

Namaste,

harmony willow

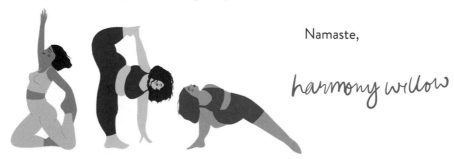

YOU ARE
STRONG
and
WORTHY

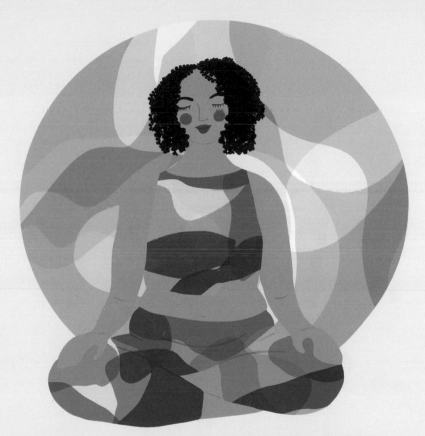

THIS IS MY HAPPY PLACE

EASY SIT
Sukhāsana

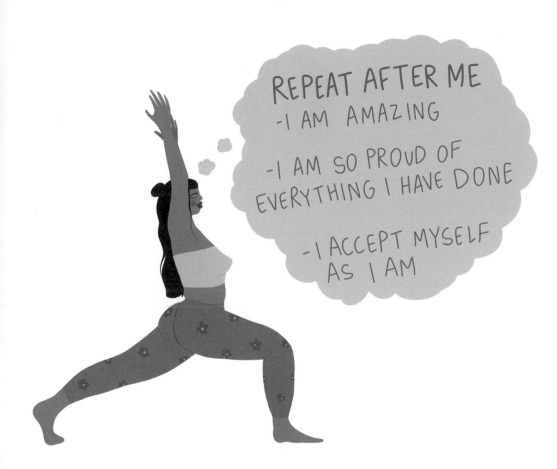

CRESCENT LUNGE
Aṣṭa Candrāsana

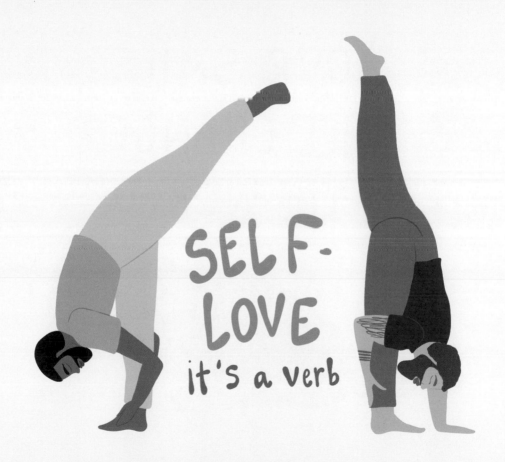

STANDING SPLITS
Ūrdhva Prasārita Eka Pādāsana

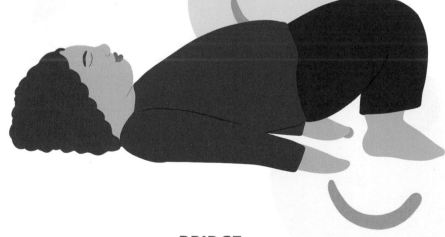

YOUR SMILE WILL CHANGE THE WORLD

BRIDGE
Setu Bandha Sarvāṅgāsana

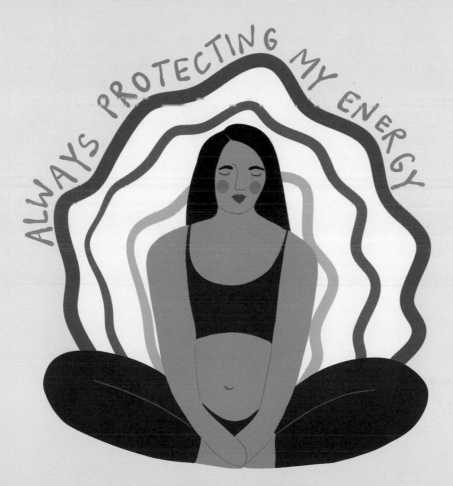

BOUND ANGLE
Baddha Koṇāsana

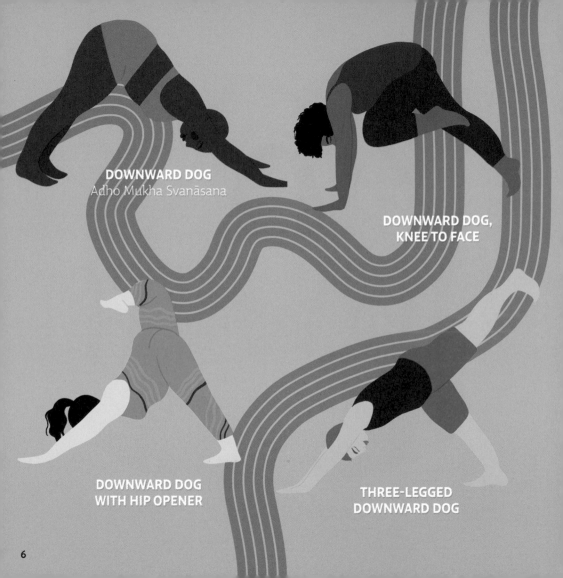

DOWNWARD DOG
Adho Mukha Svanāsana

**DOWNWARD DOG,
KNEE TO FACE**

**DOWNWARD DOG
WITH HIP OPENER**

**THREE-LEGGED
DOWNWARD DOG**

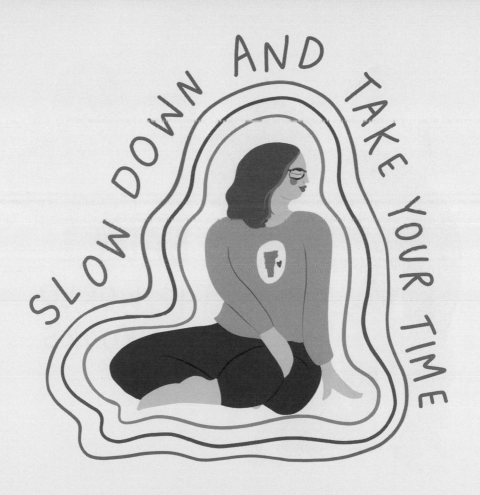

SEATED SPINAL TWIST
Parivrtta Sukhāsana

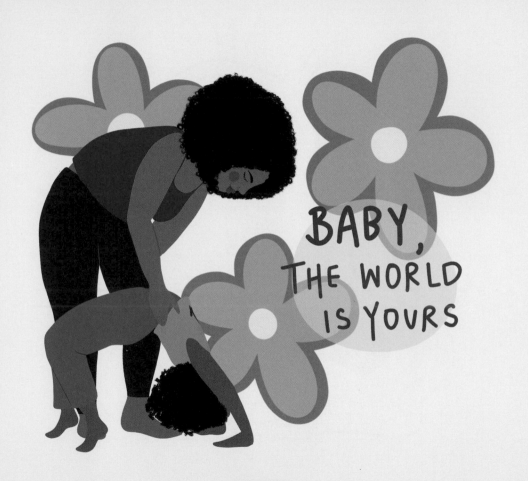

BABY, THE WORLD IS YOURS

WHEEL
Chakrāsana

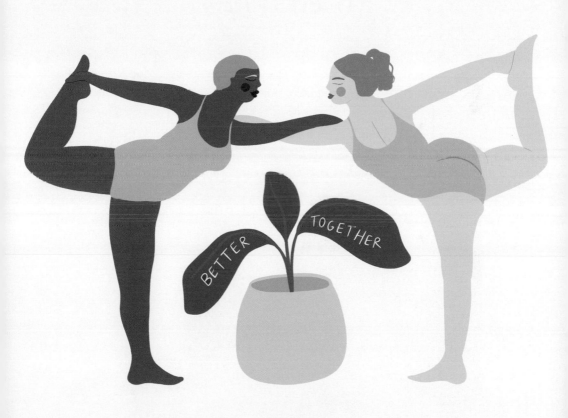

FRIENDSHIP LINK

MY GIFT TO MYSELF IS KINDNESS

CHILD'S POSE
Bālāsana

COW
Bitilāsana

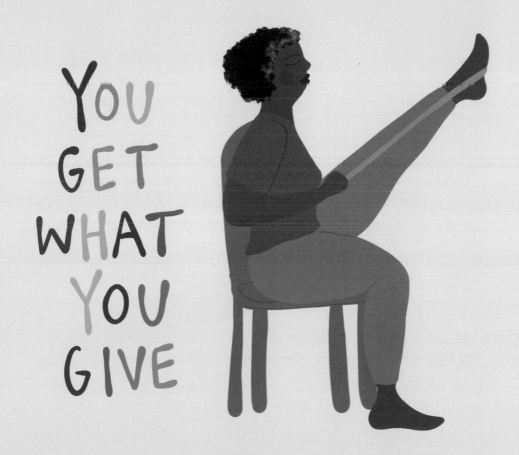

YOU GET WHAT YOU GIVE

KNEE EXTENSION

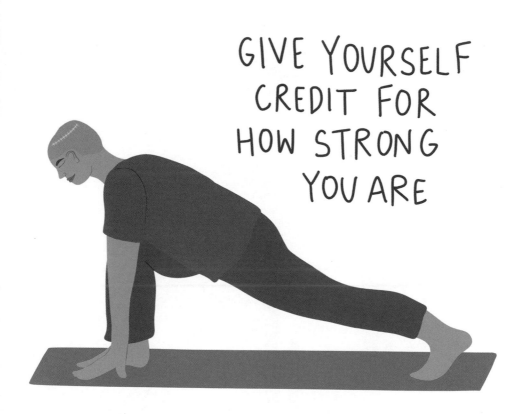

GIVE YOURSELF
CREDIT FOR
HOW STRONG
YOU ARE

LUNGE
Utthita Ashwa Sanchalanasana

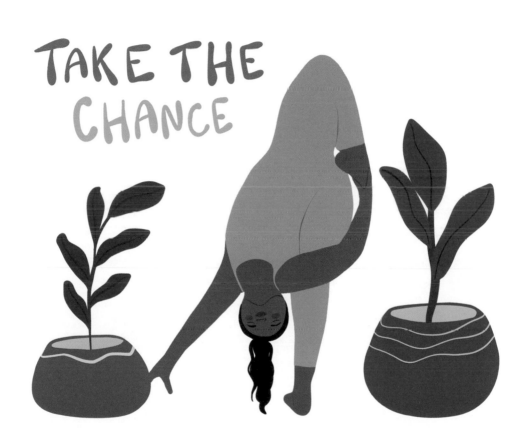

SUPER SOLDIER
Viparita Parivrtta Surya Yantrasana

gentle reminder to BREATHE

SEATED GODDESS
Utkata Koṇāsana

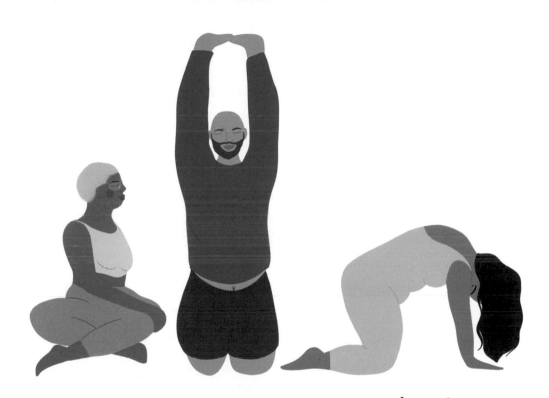

before you meditate
STRETCH it OUT

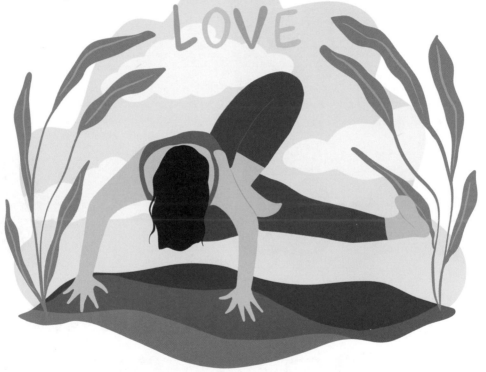

GRASSHOPPER
Maksilanagāsana

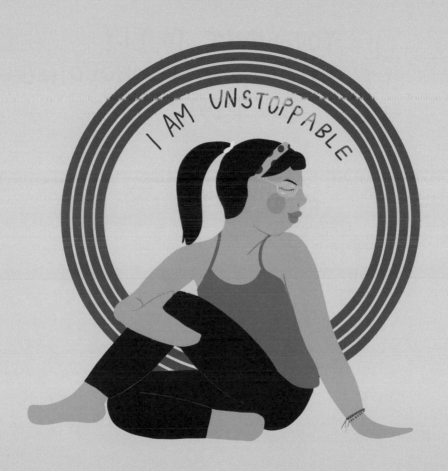

HALF LORD OF THE FISHES
Ardha Matsyendrāsana

IF YOU WANT TO FLY—
LET GO OF WHAT'S HOLDING
YOU DOWN

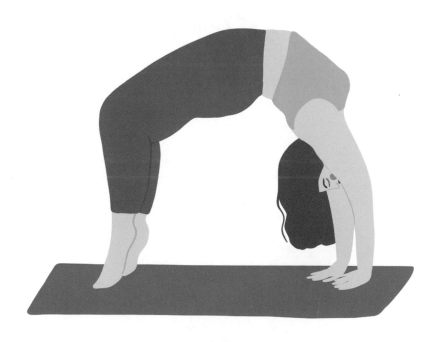

WHEEL
Ūrdhva Dhanurāsana

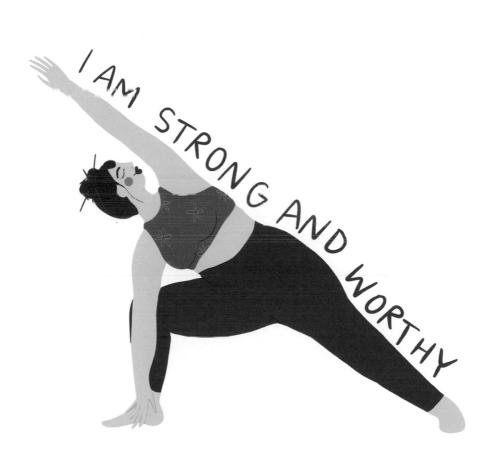

I AM STRONG AND WORTHY

EXALTED WARRIOR
Viparita Vīrabhadrāsana

I AM WHERE I NEED TO BE

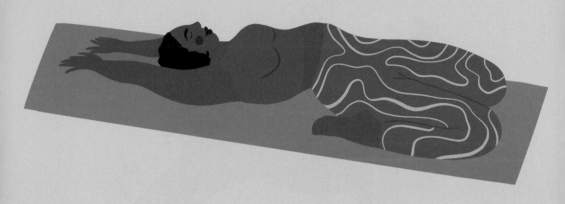

EXTENDED SUPINE HERO
Utthita Supta Virāsana

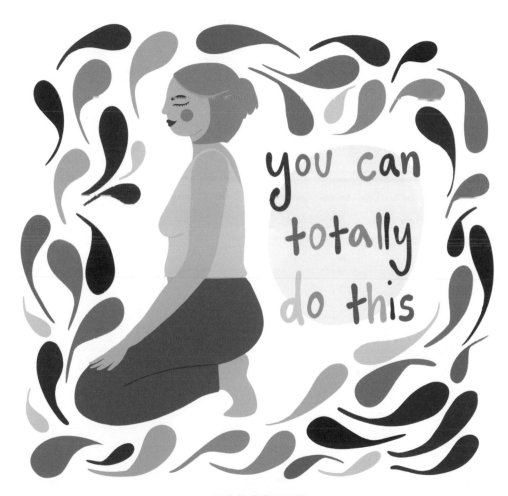

TOE SQUAT

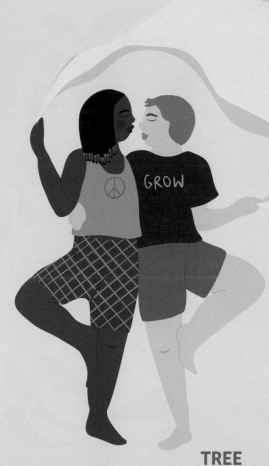

i Like you for you

TREE
Vṛkṣāsana

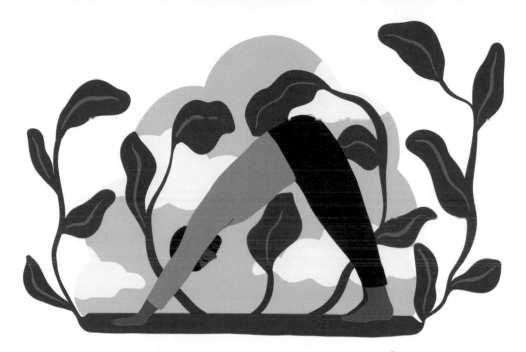

ALL THINGS CHANGE
AND WE CHANGE
WITH THEM

DOWNWARD DOG
Adho Mukha Śvanāsana

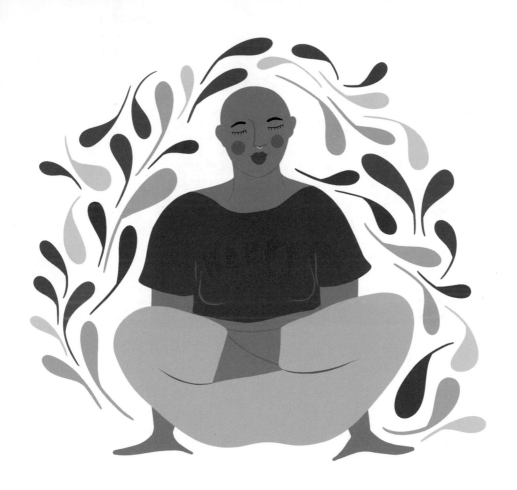

SCALE
Tolāsana, Utplutih

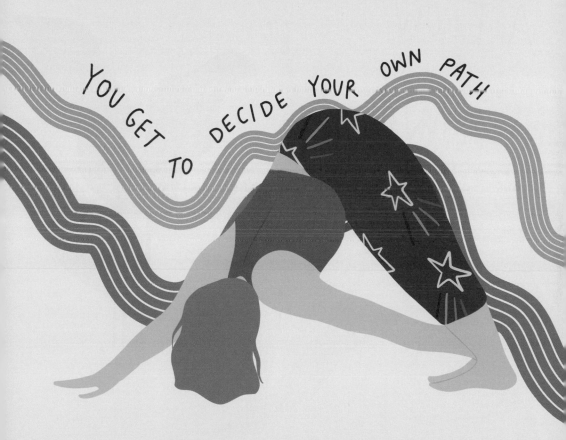

YOU GET TO DECIDE YOUR OWN PATH

REVOLVED DOWNWARD DOG
Parivṛtta Adho Mukha Svanāsana

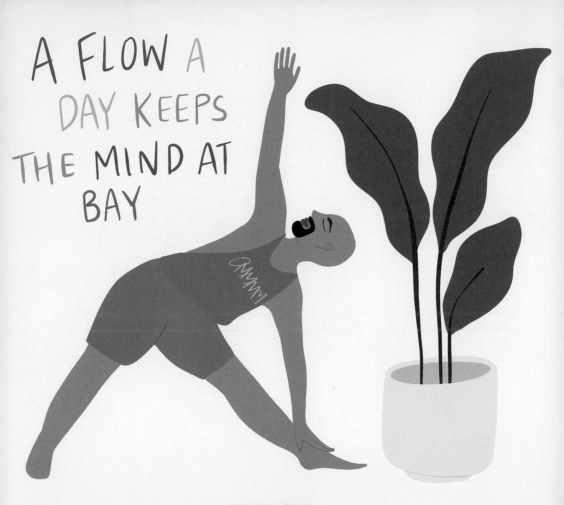

A FLOW A DAY KEEPS THE MIND AT BAY

TRIANGLE
Trikoṇāsana

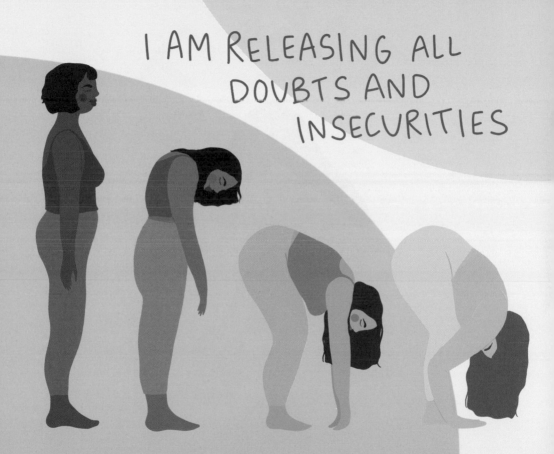

I AM RELEASING ALL DOUBTS AND INSECURITIES

STANDING ROLL DOWN

TAKE IT

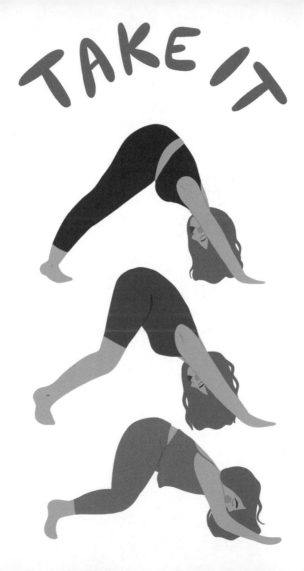

EASY

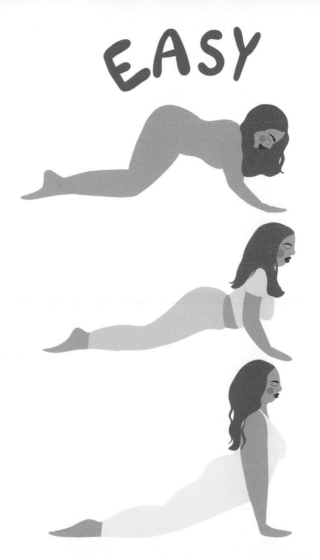

I AM WHERE I NEED TO BE

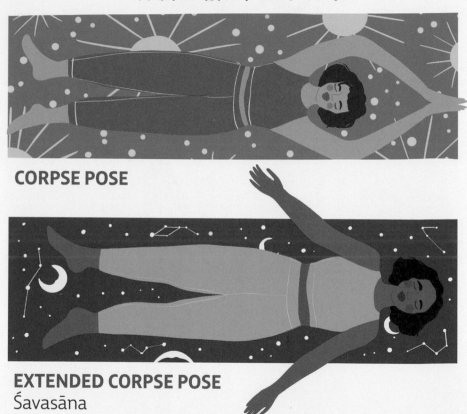

CORPSE POSE

EXTENDED CORPSE POSE
Śavasāna

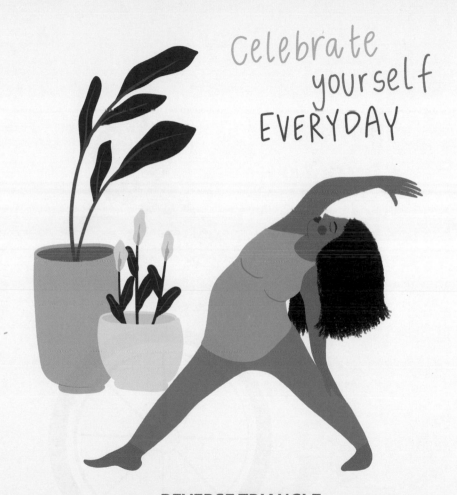

Celebrate yourself EVERYDAY

REVERSE TRIANGLE
Viparita Trikoṇāsana

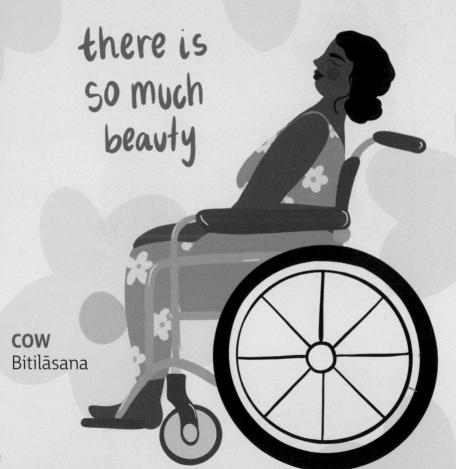

there is
so much
beauty

COW
Bitilāsana

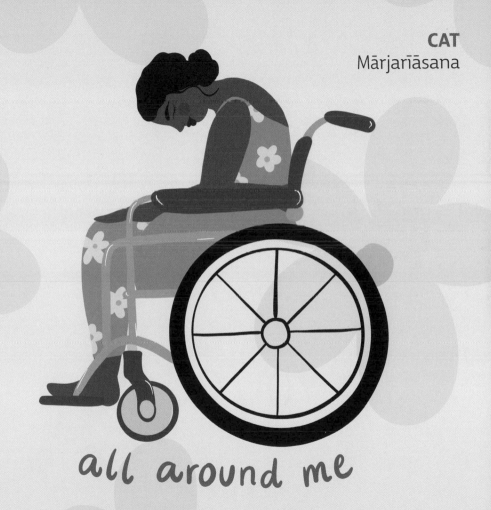

all around me

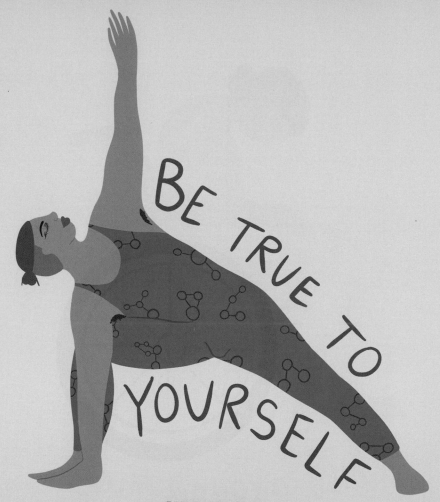

BE TRUE TO YOURSELF

SIDE ANGLE
Pārśvakonāsana

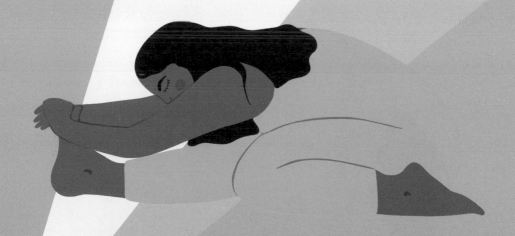

I VIBRATE POSITIVE ENERGY

SEATED THREE-LIMBED FORWARD BEND
Triaṅga Mukhaikapāda Paschimottānāsana

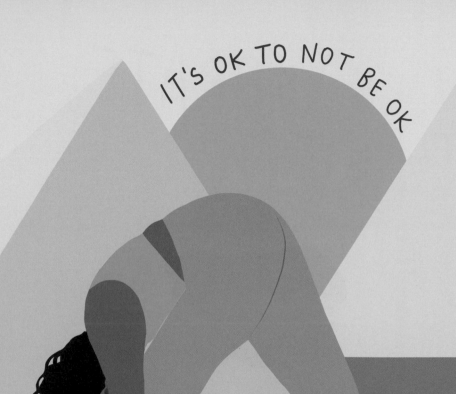

IT'S OK TO NOT BE OK

PYRAMID
Pārśottānāsana

36

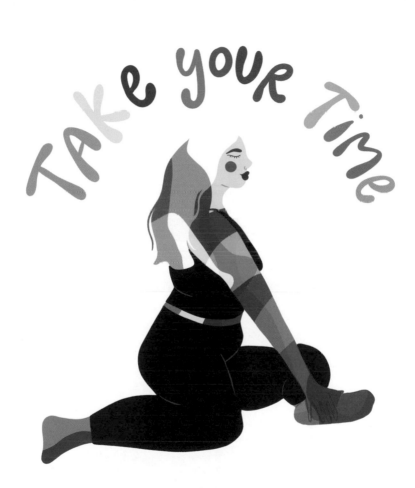

Take your Time

90/90

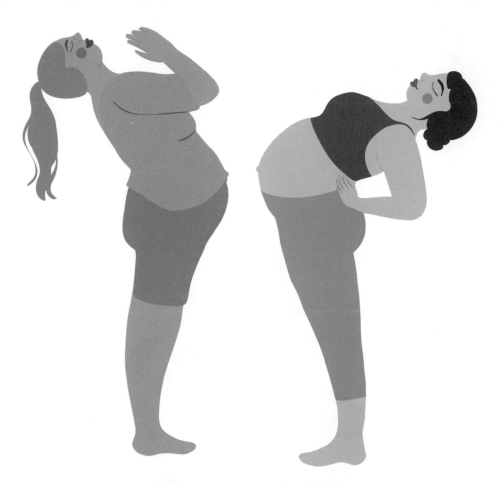

STANDING BACK BEND
Anuvittasana

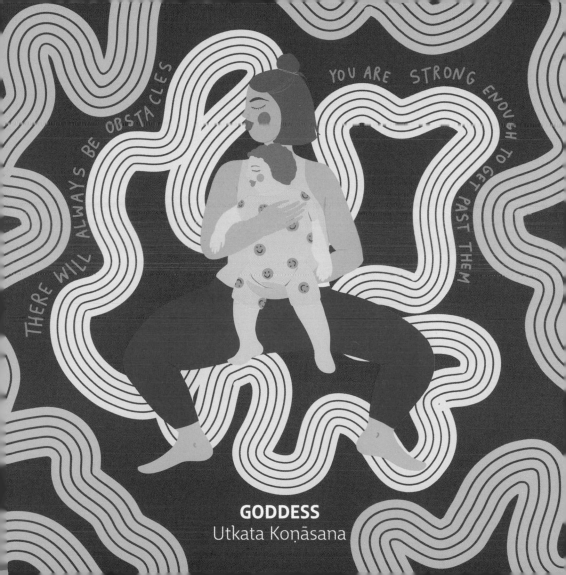

THERE WILL ALWAYS BE OBSTACLES

YOU ARE STRONG ENOUGH TO GET PAST THEM

GODDESS
Utkata Koṇāsana

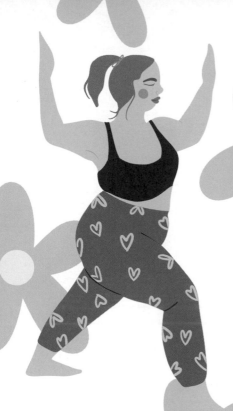

you
are valved
and
loved

WARRIOR I
Vīrabhadrāsana I

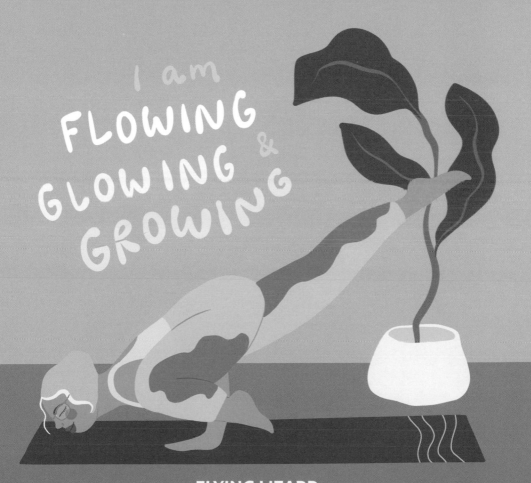

FLYING LIZARD
Utthan Pristhāsana

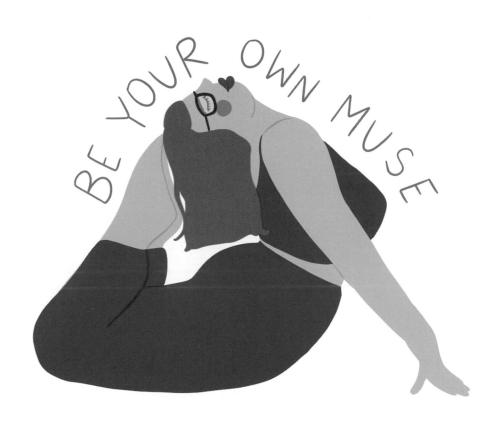

BE YOUR OWN MUSE

KING COBRA
Rāja Bhujaṅgasāna

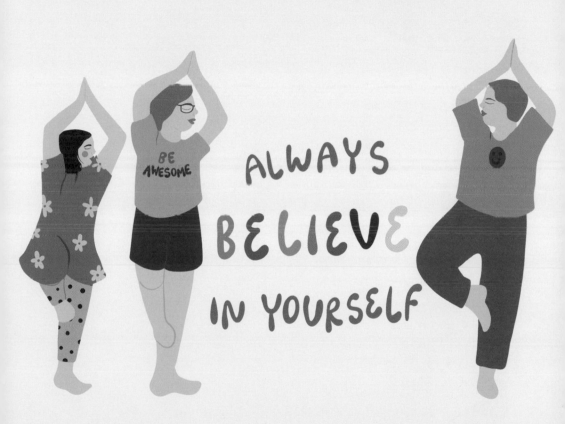

ALWAYS BELIEVE IN YOURSELF

THREE LITTLE TREES
Vṛkṣāsana

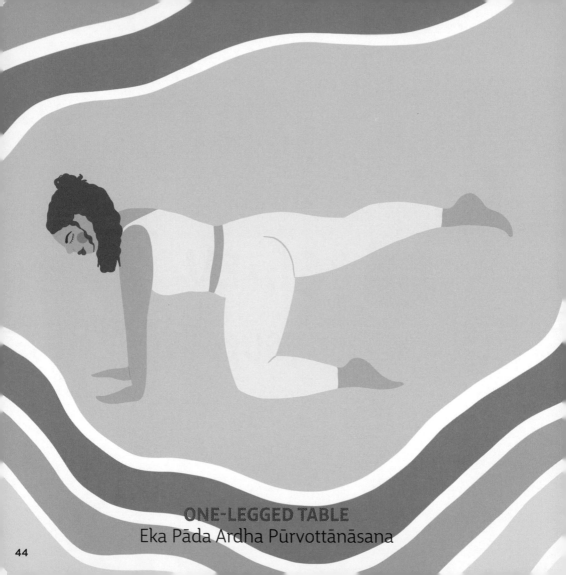

ONE-LEGGED TABLE
Eka Pāda Ardha Pūrvottānāsana

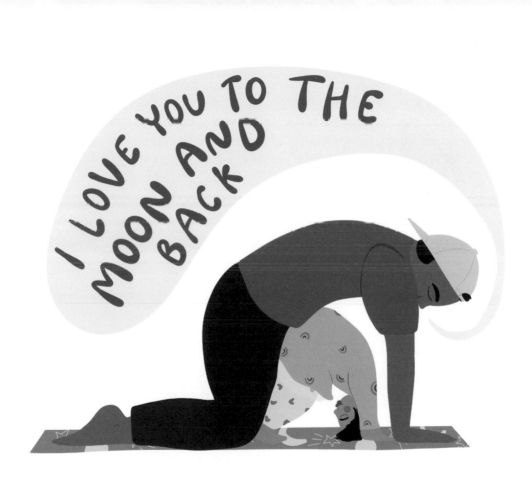

CAT
Mārjarīāsana

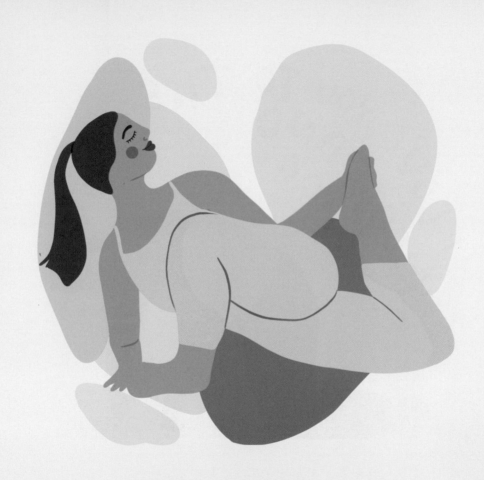

HALF TWISTED LIZARD
Parivṛtta Utthan Pristhāsana

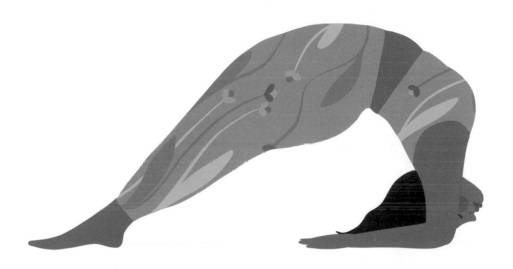

MY INTUITION IS ALWAYS ON MY SIDE

INVERTED STAFF
Dvi Pāda Viparīta Daṇḍāsana

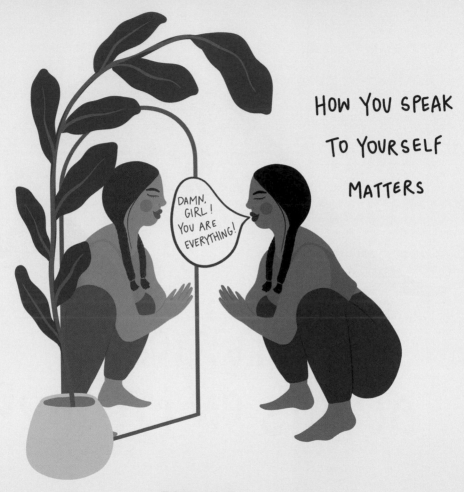

GARLAND
Mālāsana

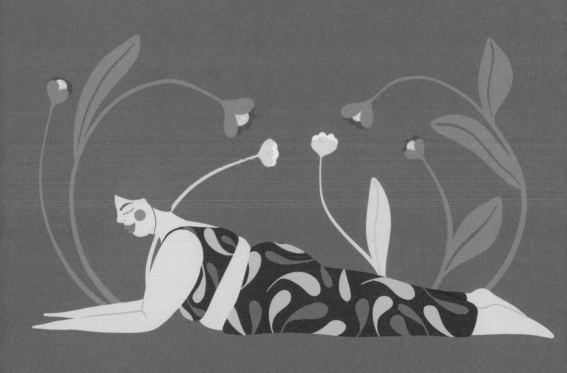

SPHINX
Sālamba Bhujaṅgāsana

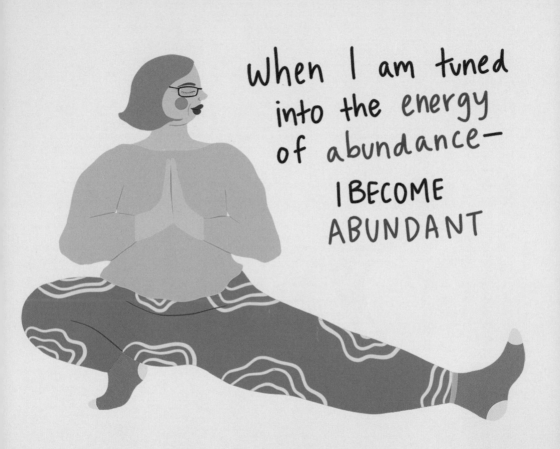

When I am tuned into the energy of abundance—

I BECOME ABUNDANT

SIDE LUNGE
Skandāsana

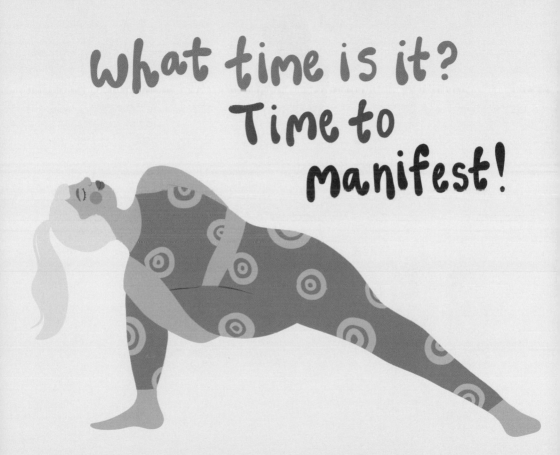

BOUND REVOLVED SIDE ANGLE
Parivṛtta Baddha Pārśvakoṇāsana

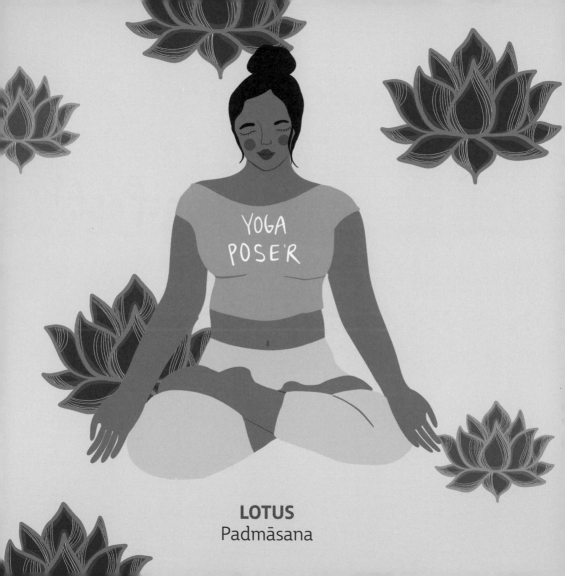

LOTUS
Padmāsana

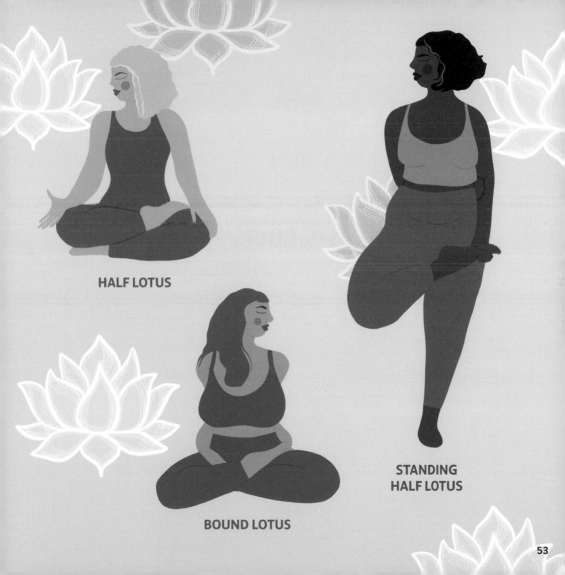

HALF LOTUS

BOUND LOTUS

STANDING
HALF LOTUS

53

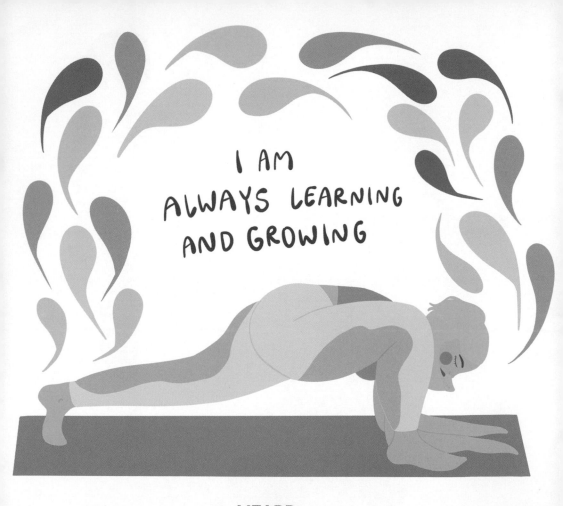

LIZARD
Vttāna Pristhāsana

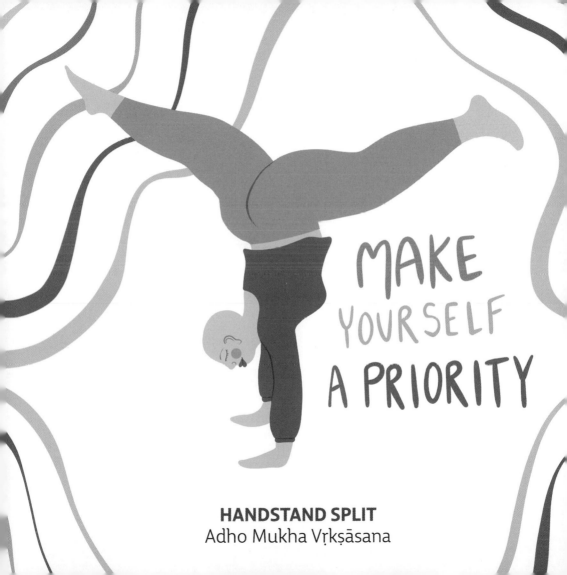

MAKE YOURSELF A PRIORITY

HANDSTAND SPLIT
Adho Mukha Vṛkṣāsana

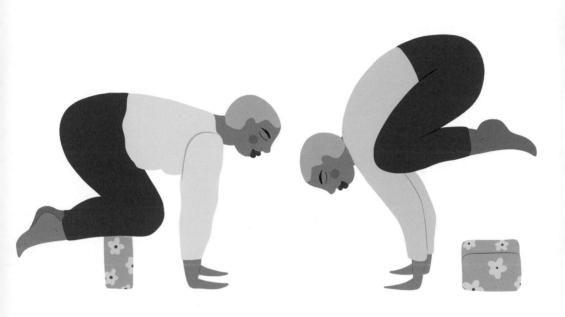

WHAT I LEARNED YESTERDAY MAKES ME STRONGER TODAY

CROW
Bakāsana

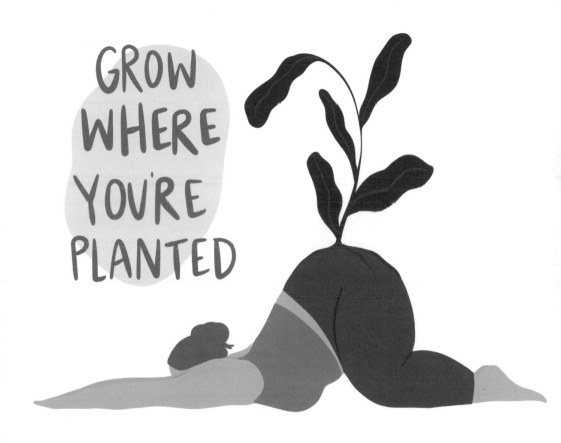

GROW WHERE YOU'RE PLANTED

EXTENDED PUPPY
Uttāna Śiśosana

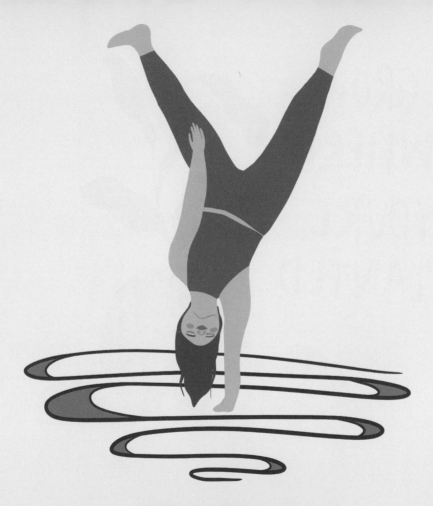

ONE-HANDED TREE
Eka Hasta Vṛkṣāsana

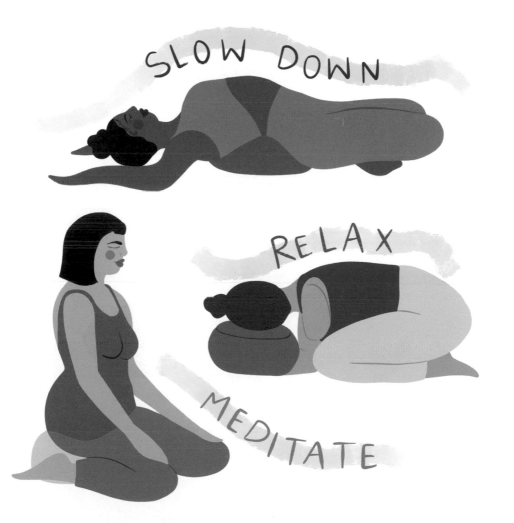

SLOW DOWN

RELAX

MEDITATE

WHATEVER YOU DECIDE TO DO IN LIFE
MAKE SURE YOU ARE HAPPY

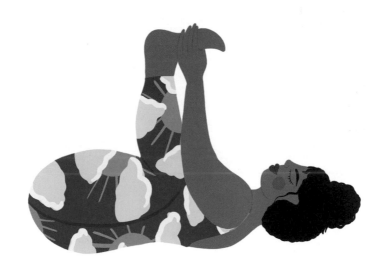

HAPPY BABY
Ānanda Bālāsana

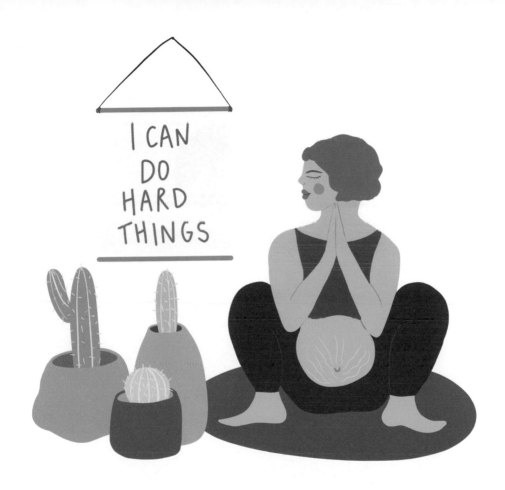

I CAN
DO
HARD
THINGS

GARLAND
Mālāsana

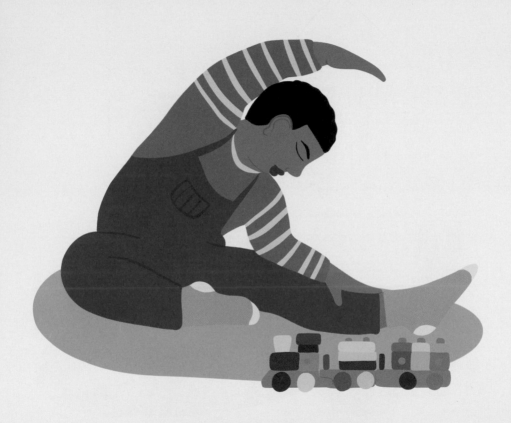

SEATED SIDE STRETCH
Parsva Upavistha Konāsana

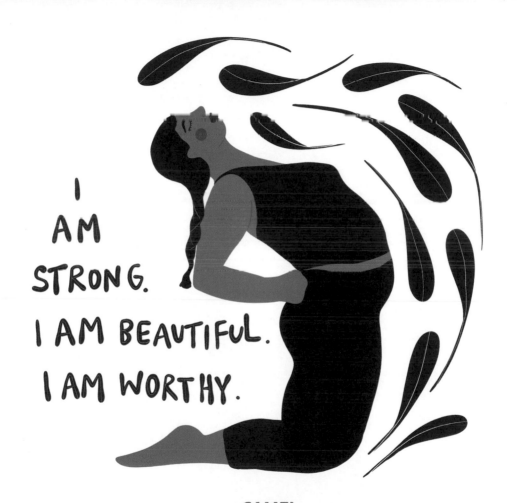

I AM STRONG.
I AM BEAUTIFUL.
I AM WORTHY.

CAMEL
Uṣṭrāsana

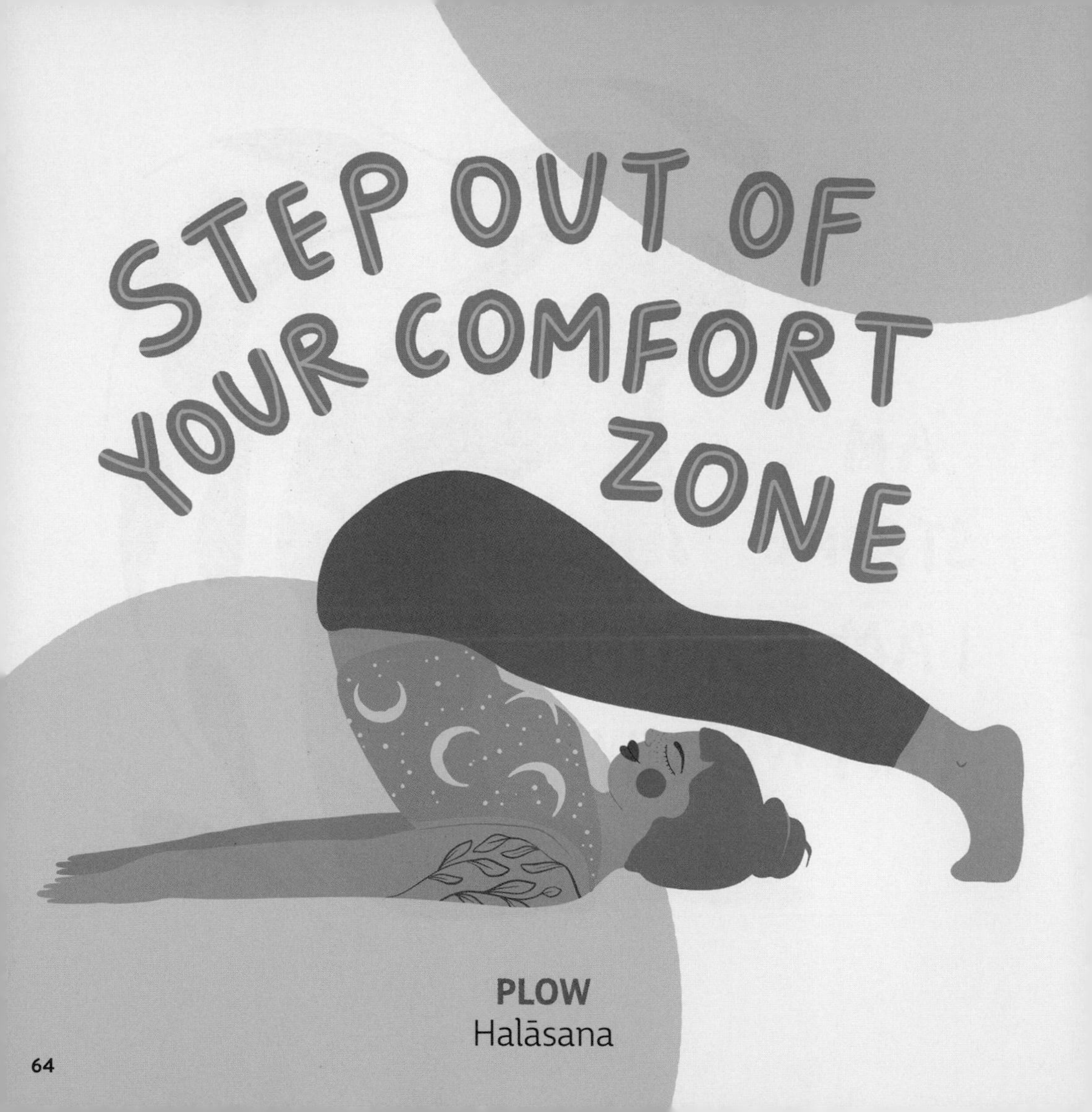

STEP OUT OF YOUR COMFORT ZONE

PLOW
Halāsana

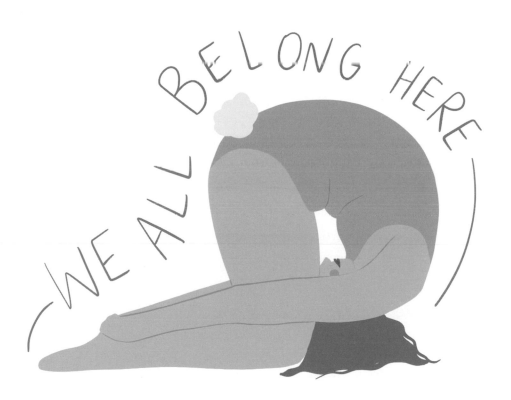

WE ALL BELONG HERE

RABBIT
Śaśankāsana

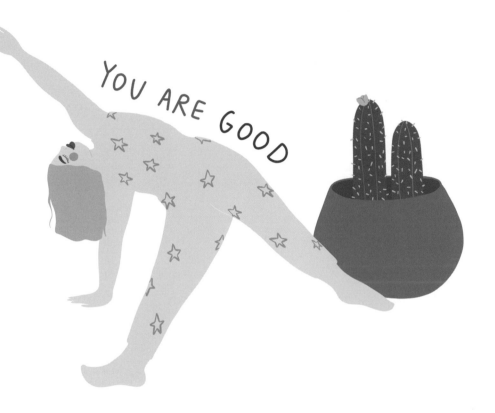

YOU ARE GOOD

FALLEN TRIANGLE
Patita Tārāsana

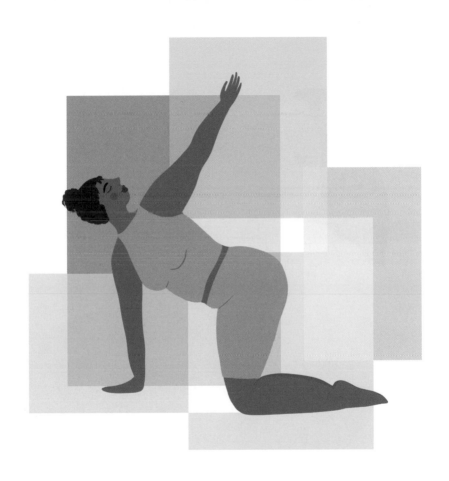

BOX, EXTENDED ARM

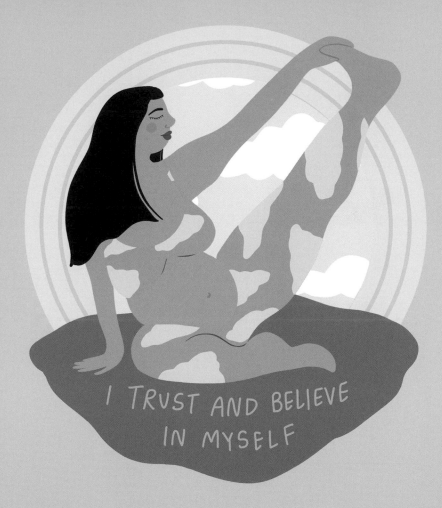

SEATED EXTENDED LEG

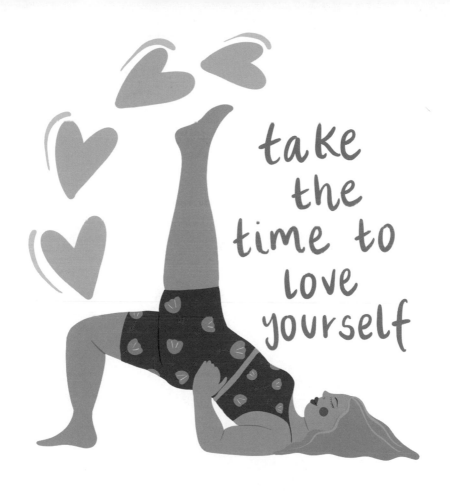

take
the
time to
love
yourself

ONE-LEGGED BRIDGE
Eka Pāda Setu Bandha Sarvāṅgāsana

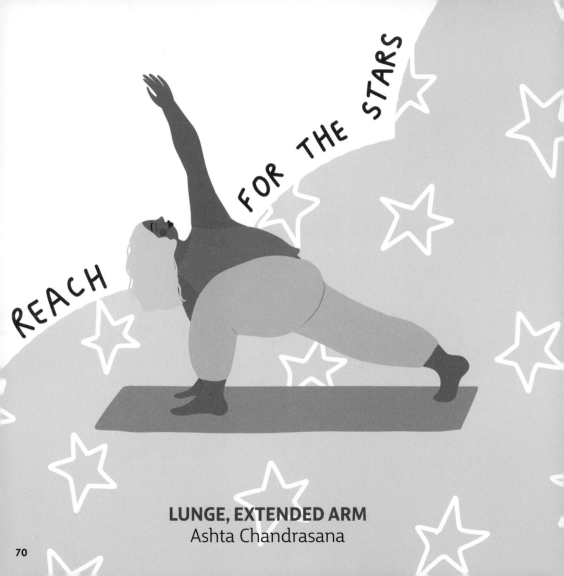

LUNGE, EXTENDED ARM
Ashta Chandrasana

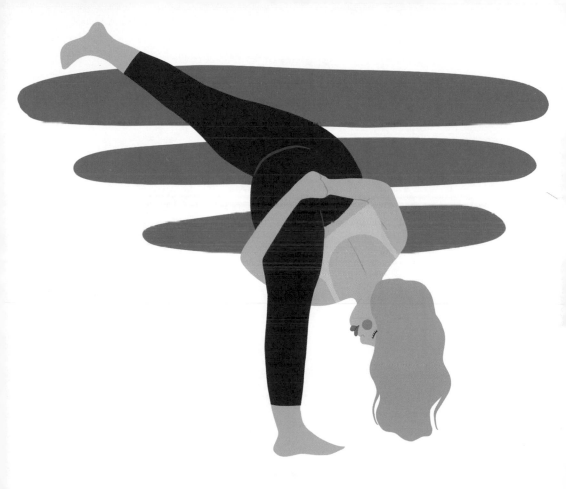

BOUND REVOLVED HALF MOON
Parivṛtta Baddha Ardha Candrāsana

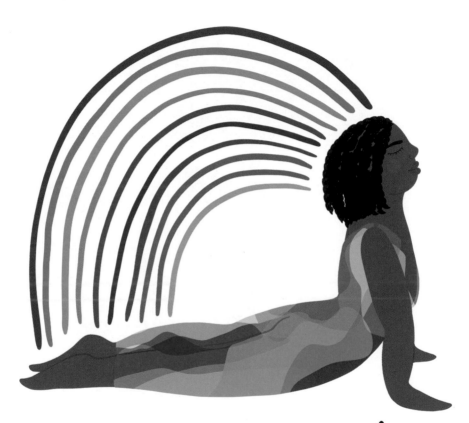

I LOVE WHO I AM
COBRA
Bhujaṅgāsana

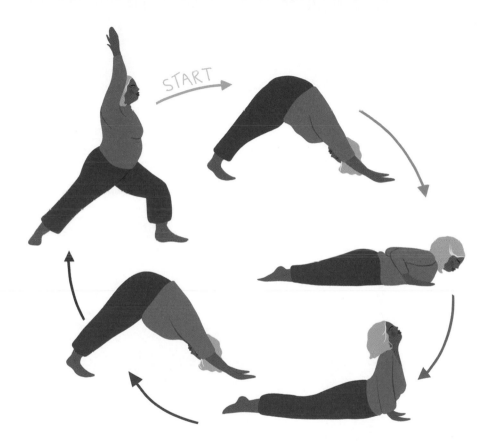

START

REFRESHING FLOW

I AM GRATEFUL FOR ALL THE BEAUTY I CREATE

DOWNWARD DOG
Adho Mukha Svanāsana

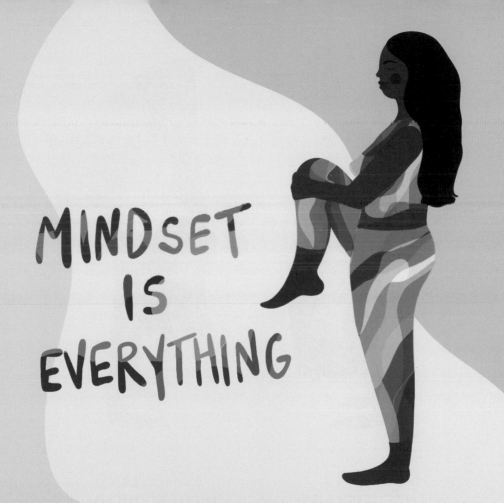

MINDSET IS EVERYTHING

STANDING KNEE TO CHEST

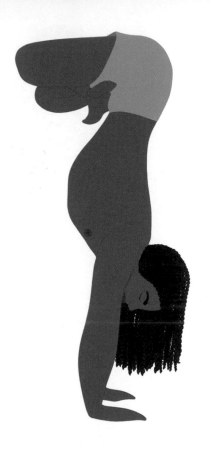

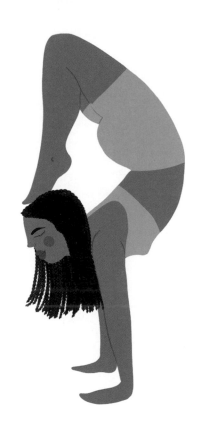

**HANDSTAND
WITH LOTUS LEGS**

**HANDSTAND
WITH SCORPION**
Vr̄śhikāsana I

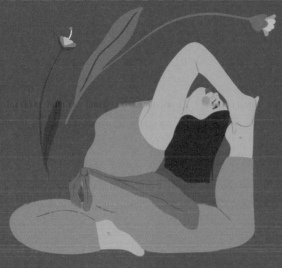

KING PIGEON

CAMEL

I AM
GRATEFUL FOR ALL
THE BEAUTIFUL SOULS
IN MY LIFE

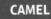

HALF BOAT

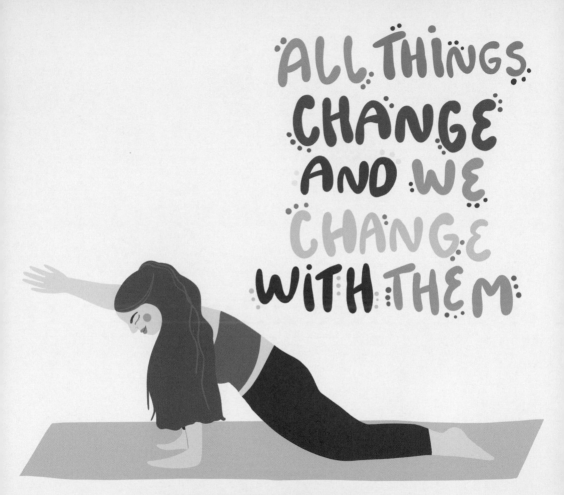

LUNGE, ARM EXTENDED

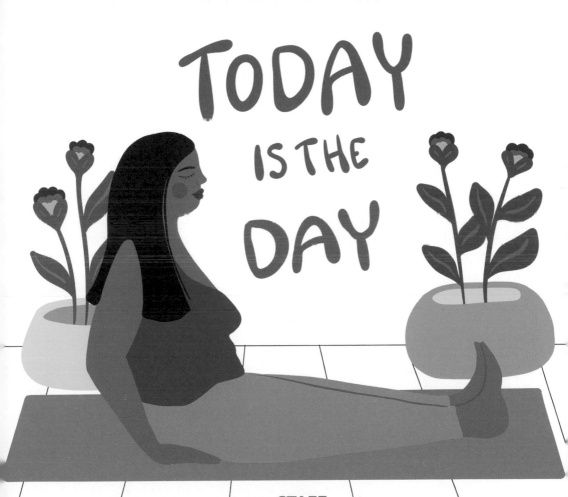

TODAY IS THE DAY

STAFF
Daṇḍāsana

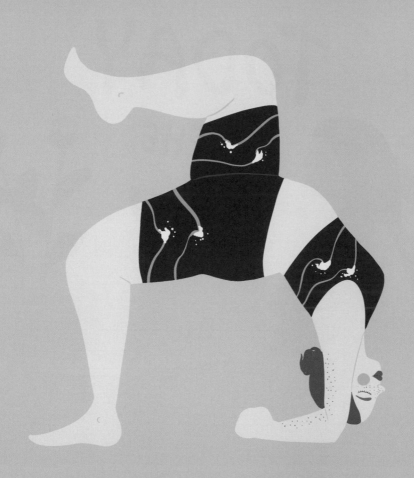

ONE-LEGGED INVERTED STAFF
Eka Pāda Viparīta Daṇḍāsana

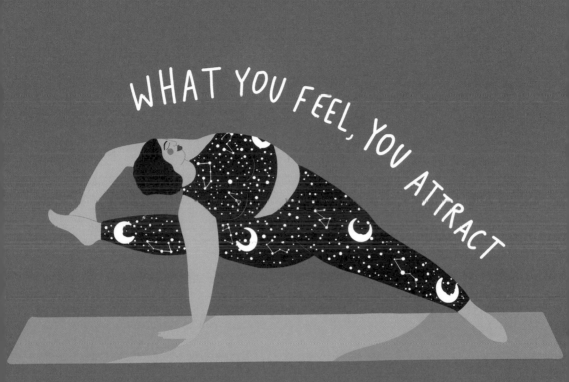

REVOLVED BIRD OF PARADISE
Parivṛtta Svarga Dvijāsana

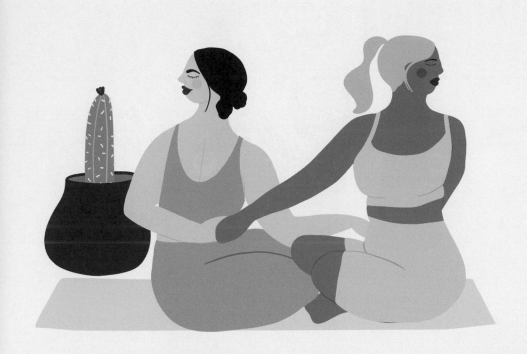

GENTLE PARTNER TWIST

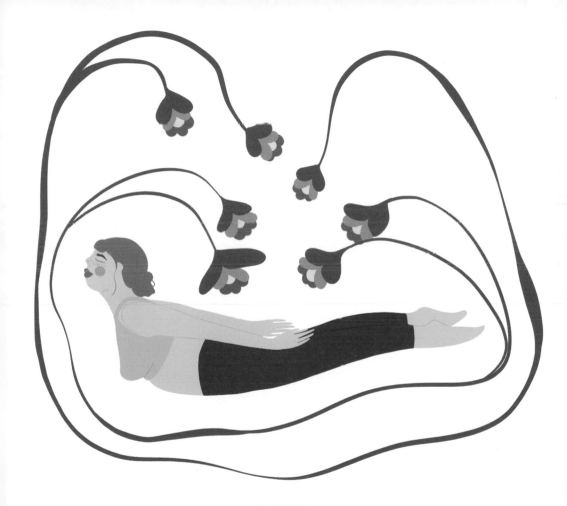

LOCUST
Śalabhāsana

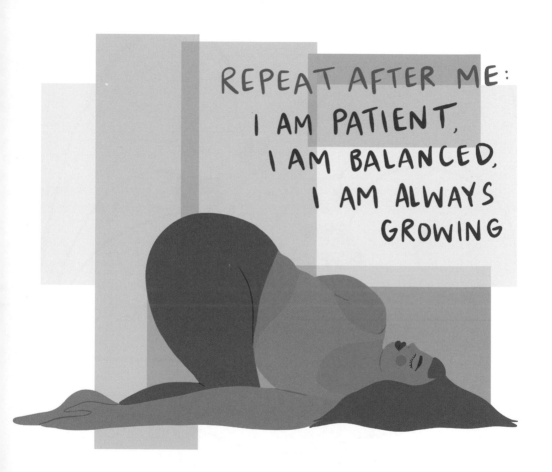

REVOLVED CHILD'S POSE
Pārśva Bālāsana

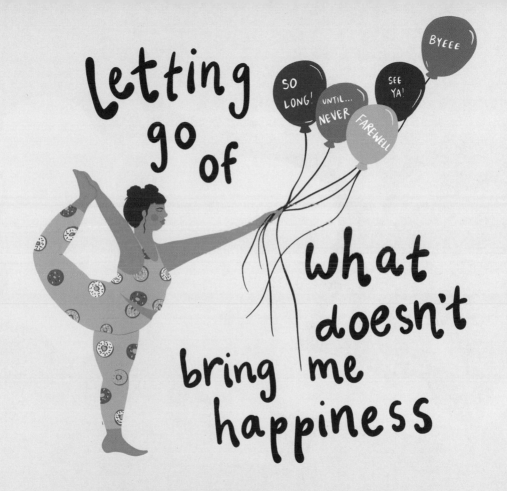

letting go of what doesn't bring me happiness

LORD OF THE DANCE
Parivrtta Naṭarājāsana

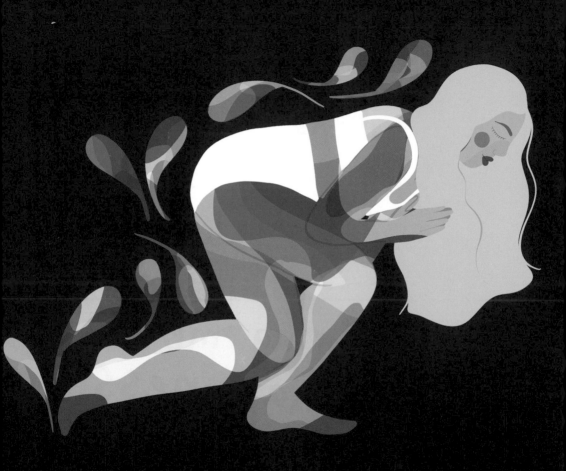

SHIVA SQUAT

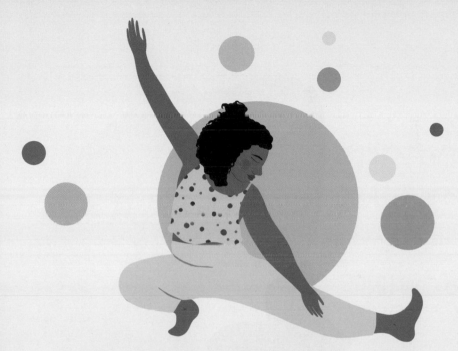

WHETHER I SUCCEED OR FAIL,
I LEARN FROM MY EXPERIENCES.

SIDE LUNGE, ARMS EXTENDED
Skandāsana

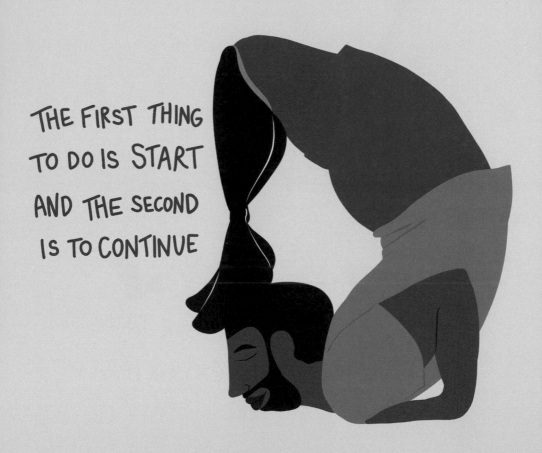

THE FIRST THING TO DO IS START AND THE SECOND IS TO CONTINUE

FORMIDABLE FACE
Ganda Bherundāsana

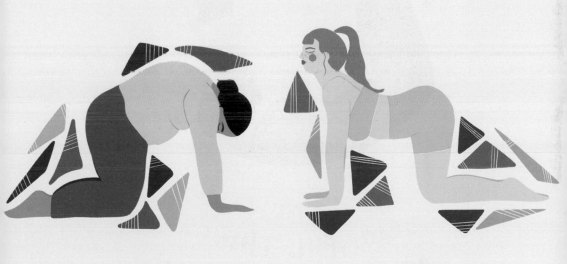

CAT
Mārjarīāsana

COW
Bitilāsana

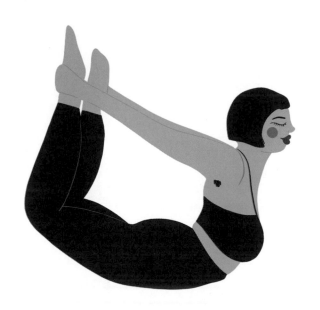

I KNOW
BEAUTIFUL THINGS
ARE ABOUT TO HAPPEN

BOW
Dhanurāsāna

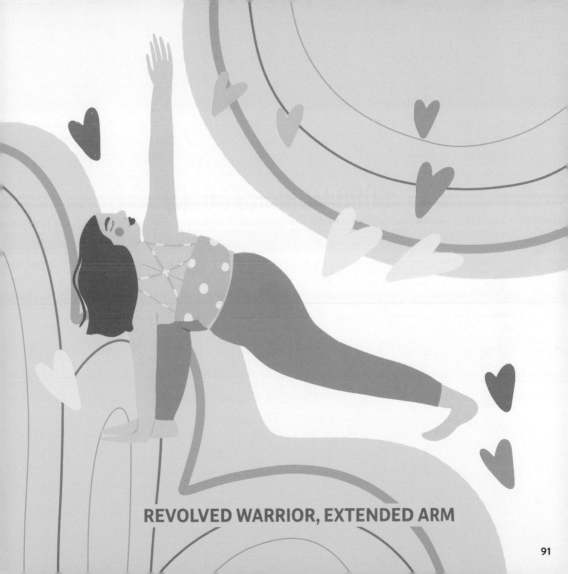

REVOLVED WARRIOR, EXTENDED ARM

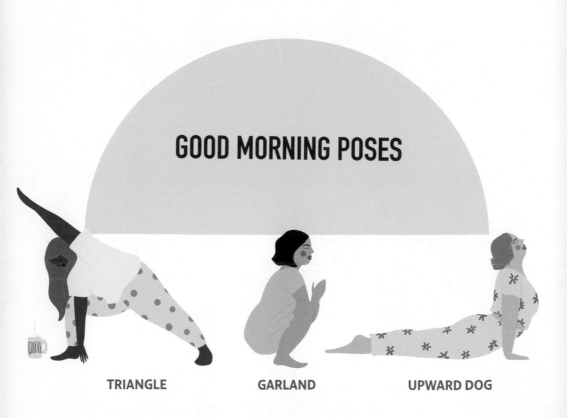

GOOD MORNING POSES

TRIANGLE   GARLAND   UPWARD DOG

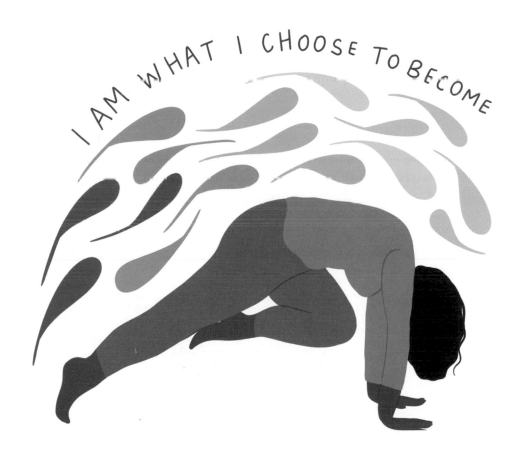

I AM WHAT I CHOOSE TO BECOME

KNEE TO ELBOW
Phalakāsana I

93

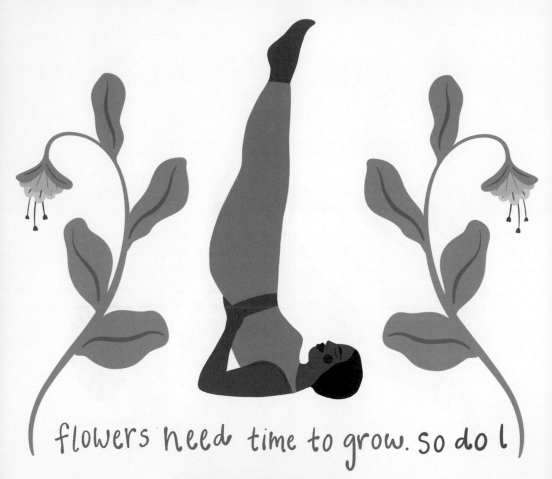

flowers need time to grow. so do I

SHOULDER STAND
Sarvāṅgāsana

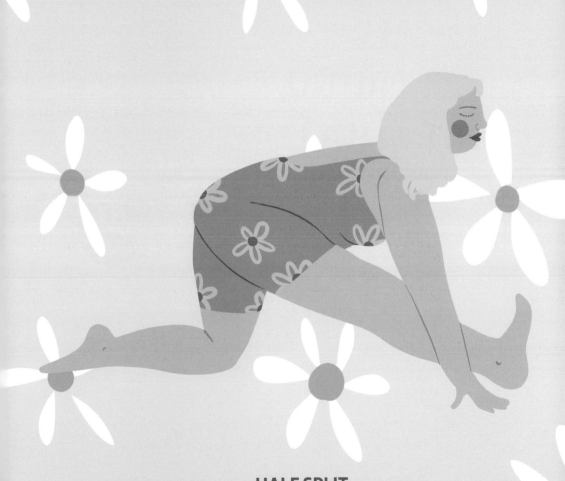

HALF SPLIT
Ardha Hanumānāsana

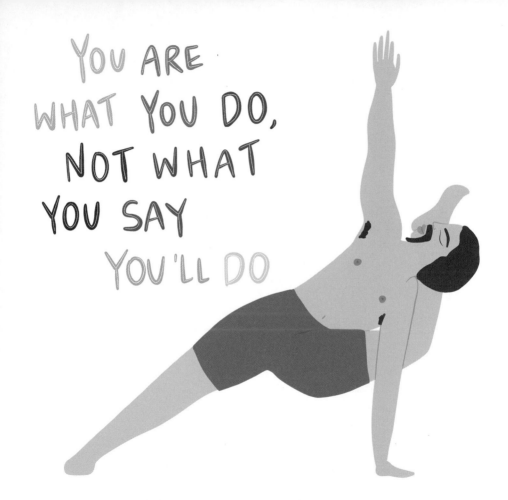

YOU ARE WHAT YOU DO, NOT WHAT YOU SAY YOU'LL DO

DESTROYER OF THE UNIVERSE
Bhairavāsana

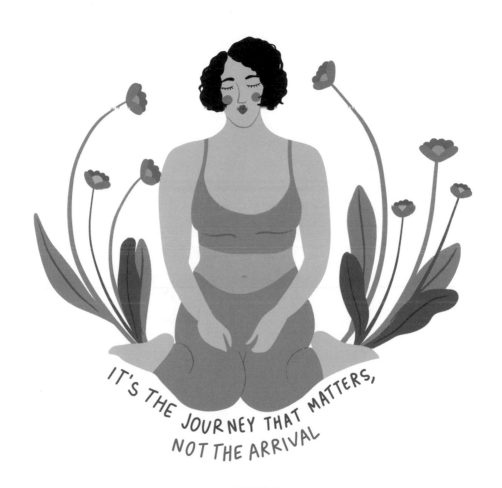

IT'S THE JOURNEY THAT MATTERS, NOT THE ARRIVAL

HERO
Virāsana

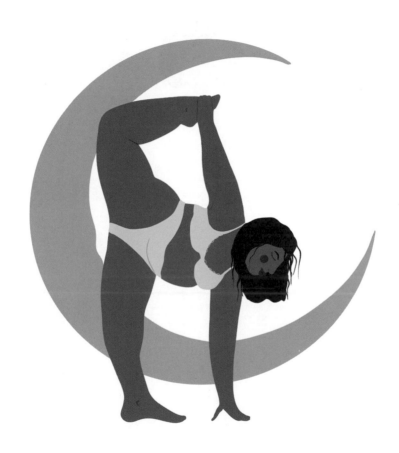

SUGARCANE
Ardha Candra Cāpāsana

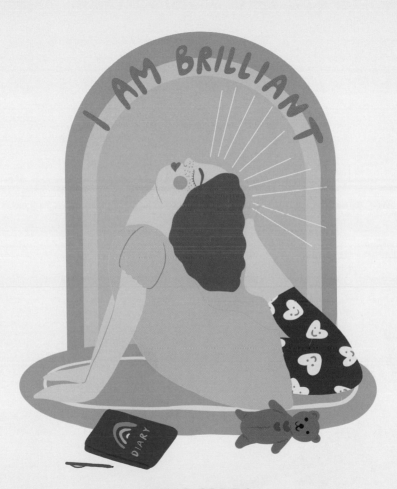

KING COBRA
Rāja Bhujaṅgāsana

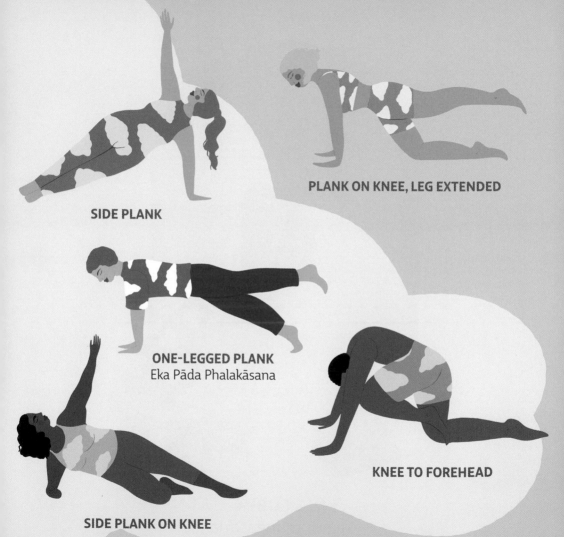

SIDE PLANK

PLANK ON KNEE, LEG EXTENDED

ONE-LEGGED PLANK
Eka Pāda Phalakāsana

KNEE TO FOREHEAD

SIDE PLANK ON KNEE

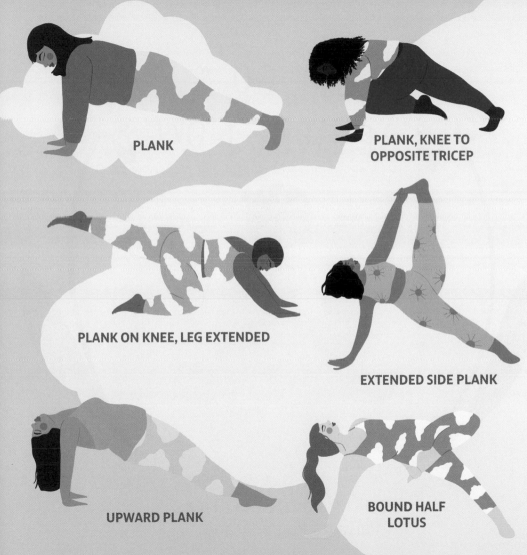

PLANK

PLANK, KNEE TO
OPPOSITE TRICEP

PLANK ON KNEE, LEG EXTENDED

EXTENDED SIDE PLANK

UPWARD PLANK

BOUND HALF
LOTUS

101

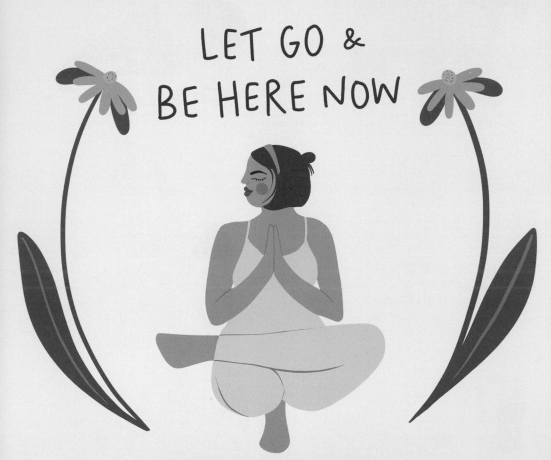

LET GO &
BE HERE NOW

SQUATTING TOE BALANCE
Parivrtta Prapadasana

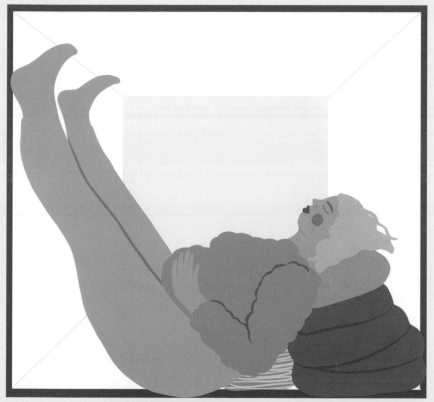

LEGS UP THE WALL
Supta Daṇḍāsana

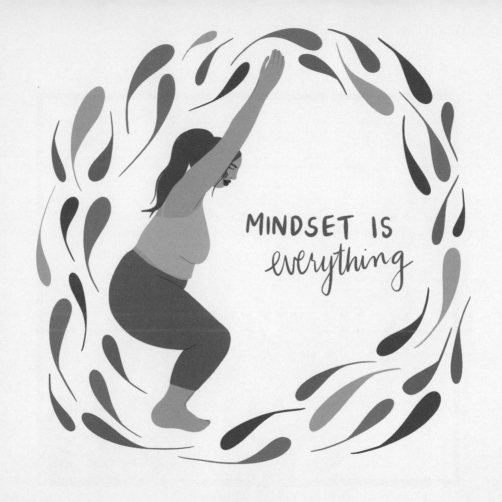

MINDSET IS *everything*

CHAIR
Utkaṭāsana

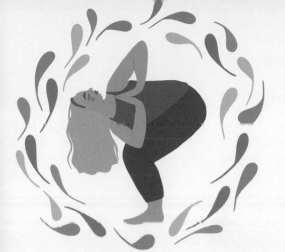

REVOLVED CHAIR

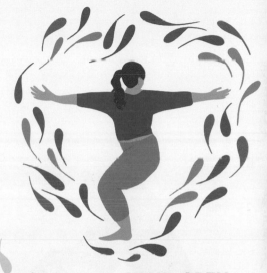

CHAIR, OPEN ARM TWIST

REVOLVED CHAIR, EXTENDED ARM

105

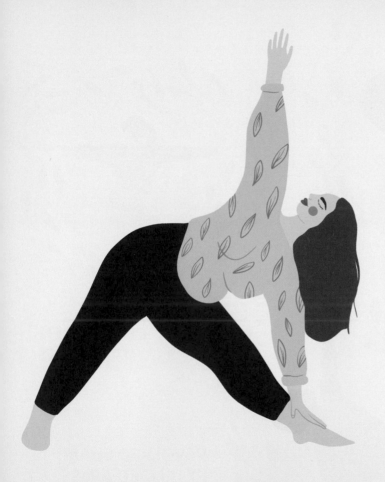

I
AM
GRATEFUL
FOR
ALL THE
SUCCESS
I'VE
EARNED

TRIANGLE
Trikoṇāsana

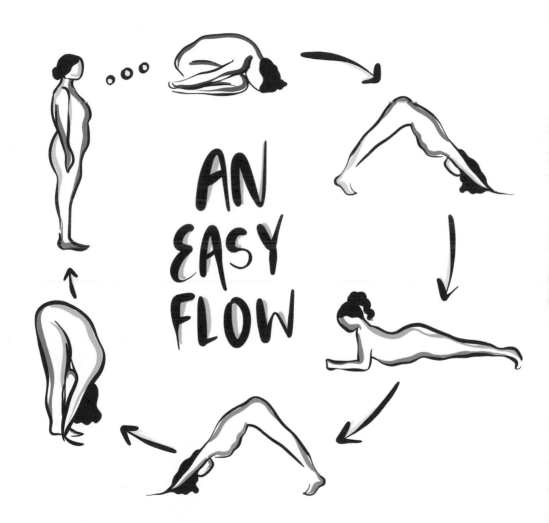

AN EASY FLOW

I AM OPEN TO THE ABUNDANCE FLOWING TO ME

EXALTED CRESCENT LUNGE
Viparita Vīrabhadrāsana

CRESCENT LUNGE
Aṣṭa Candrāsana

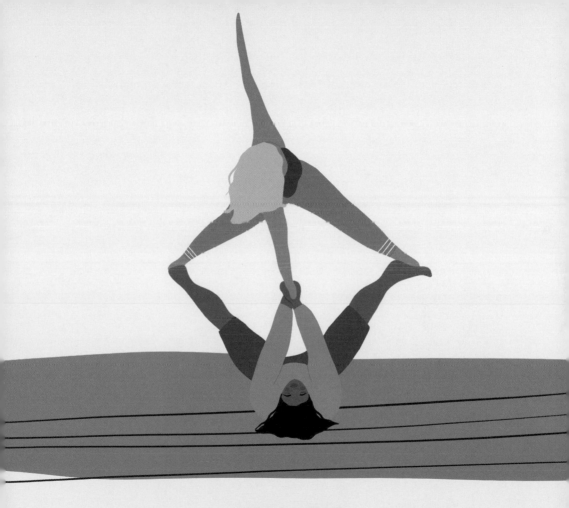

NORTH STAR
Utthita Tāḍāsana

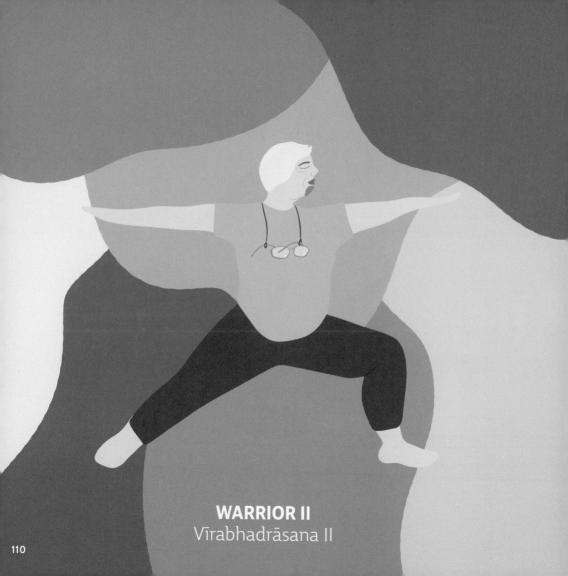

WARRIOR II
Vīrabhadrāsana II

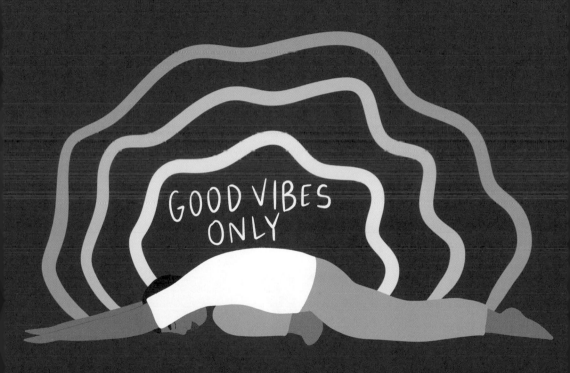

SLEEPING SWAN
Kapotāsana II

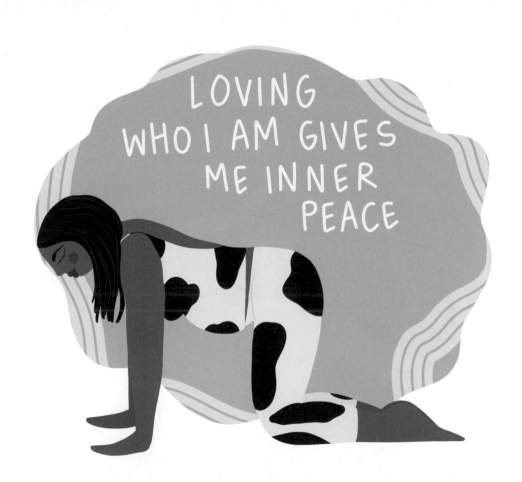

COW
Bitilāsana

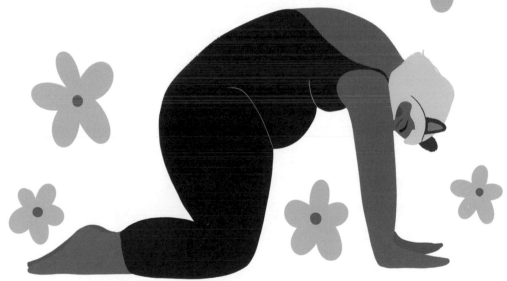

all of my hard
work is paying off

CAT
Mārjarīāsana

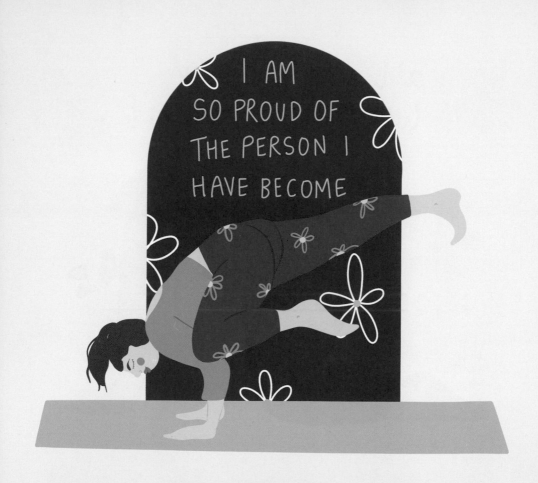

I AM
SO PROUD OF
THE PERSON I
HAVE BECOME

ONE-LEGGED CROW
Eka Pāda Kākāsana

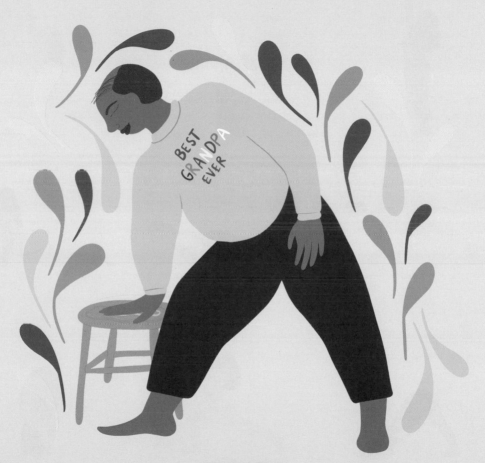

TRIANGLE
Trikoṇāsana

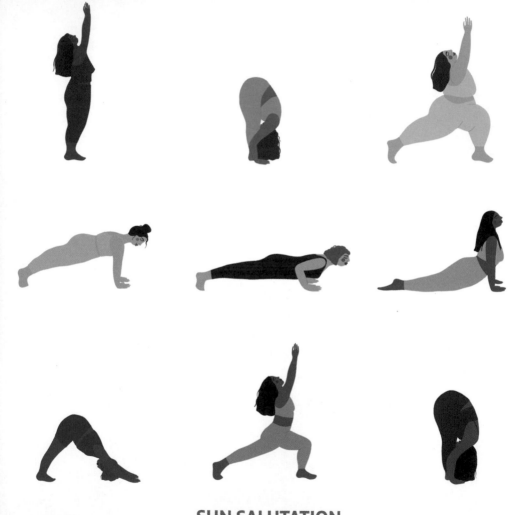

SUN SALUTATION

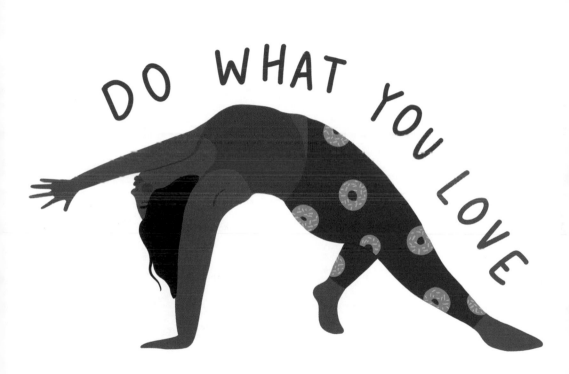

WILD THING
Camatkārāsana

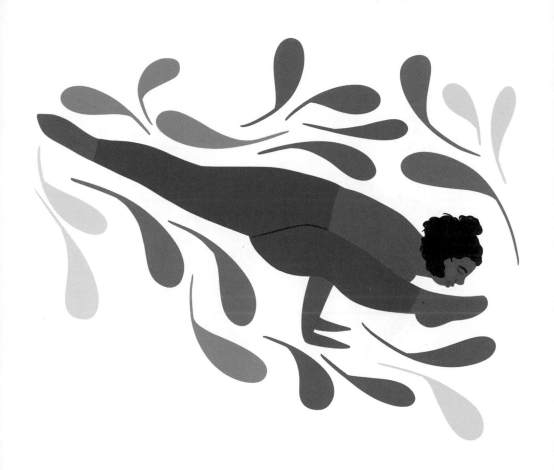

POSE DEDICATED TO THE SAGE KOUNDINYA I
Eka Pāda Koundinyāsana I

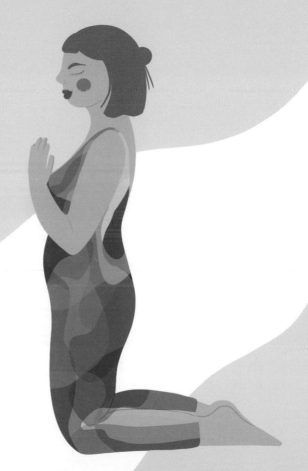

KNEELING, PRAYER HANDS

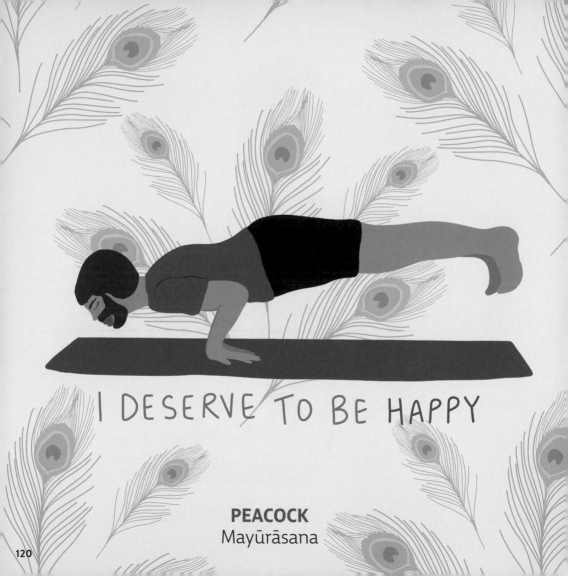

I DESERVE TO BE HAPPY

PEACOCK
Mayūrāsana

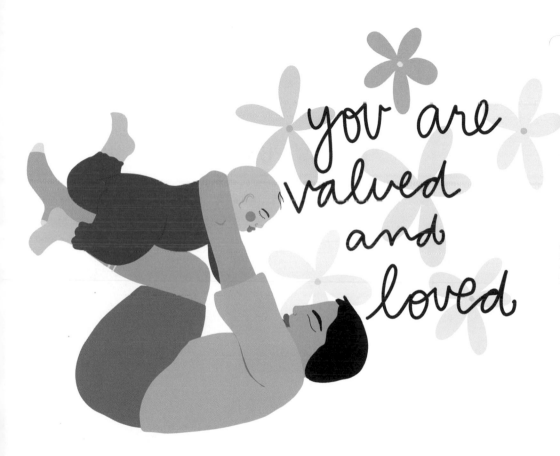

you are valued and loved

HAPPY BABY
Ānanda Bālāsana

MIDDAY POSES

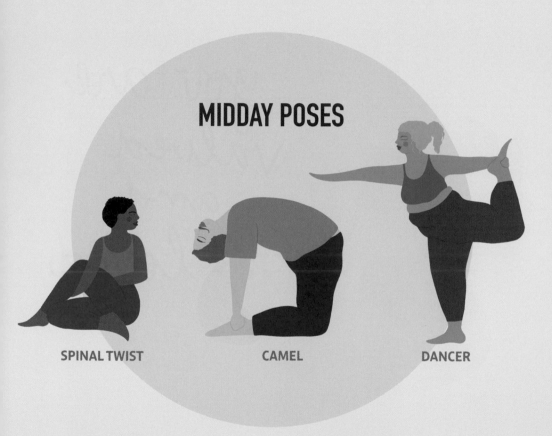

SPINAL TWIST

CAMEL

DANCER

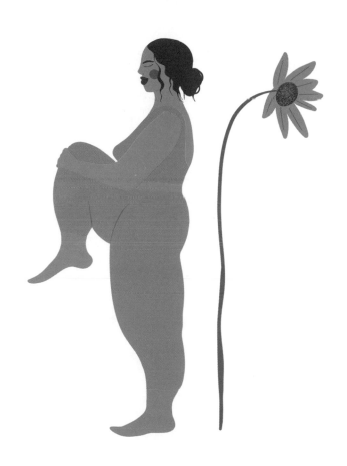

STANDING KNEE TO CHEST
Tādāsana Pavanmuktāsana

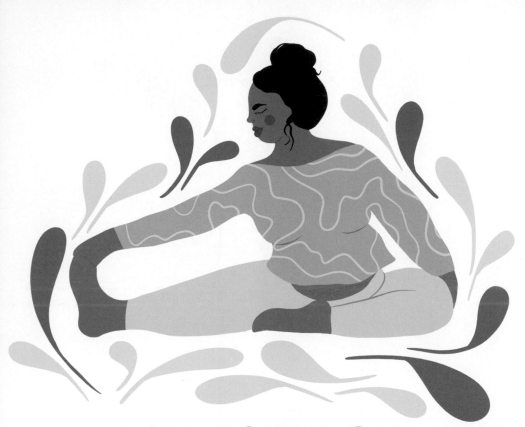

I AM BEAUTIFUL

HAND TO TOE
Utthita Hasta Pādāṅguṣṭhāsana

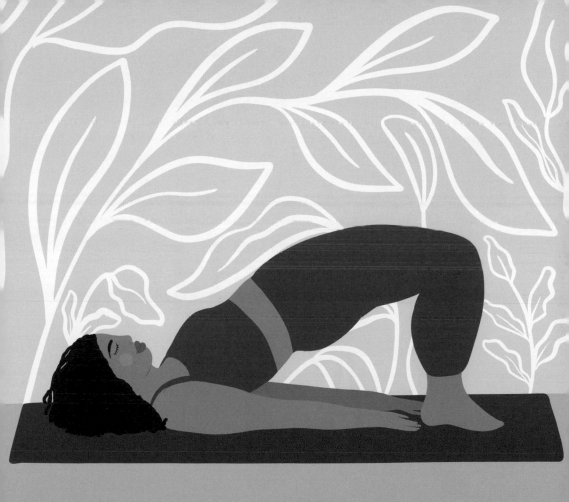

BRIDGE
Setu Bandha Sarvāṅgāsana

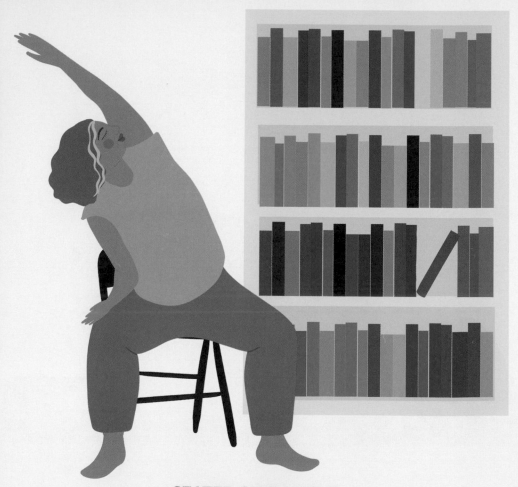

SEATED SIDE ANGLE
Utthita Pārśvakonāsana

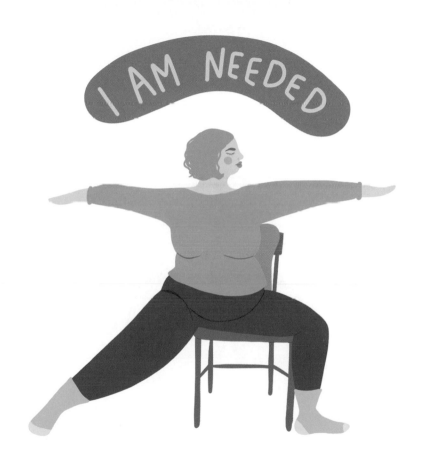

WARRIOR II WITH CHAIR
Vīrabhadrāsana II

127

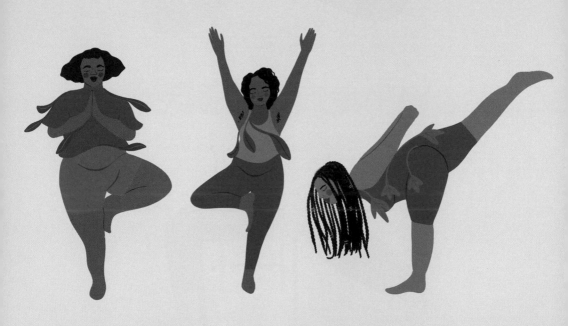

TREE
Vṛkṣāsana

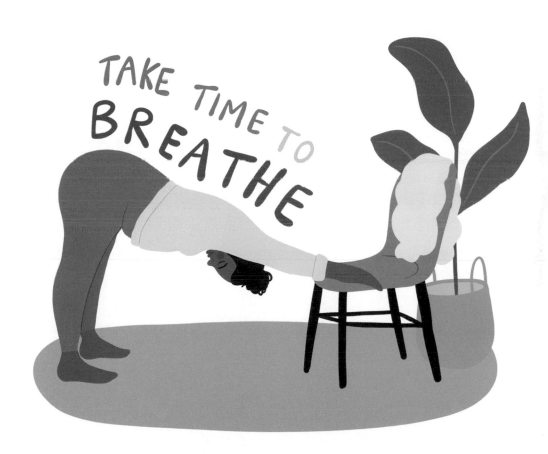

TAKE TIME TO BREATHE

DOWNWARD DOG WITH CHAIR
Adho Mukha Svanāsana

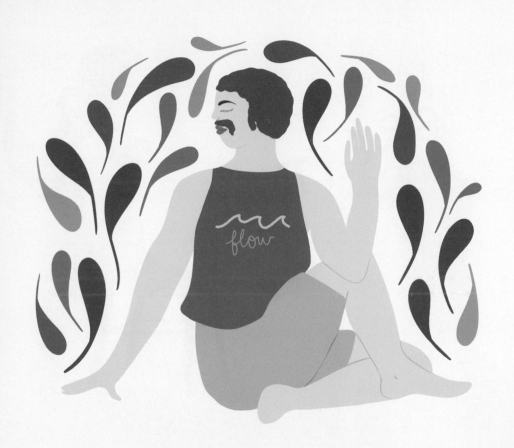

HALF LORD OF THE FISHES
Ardha Matsyendrāsana

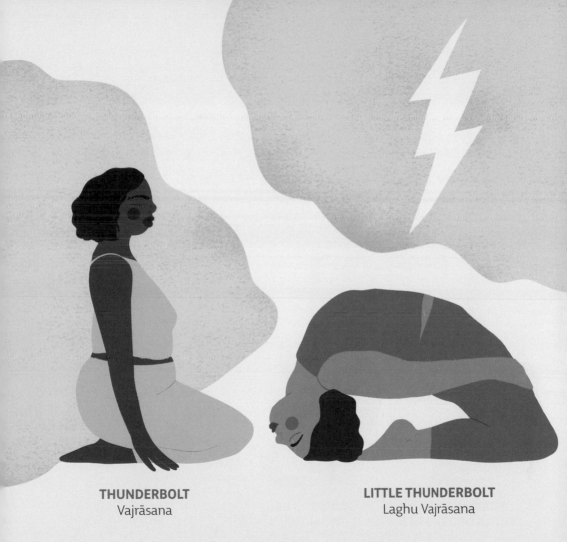

THUNDERBOLT
Vajrāsana

LITTLE THUNDERBOLT
Laghu Vajrāsana

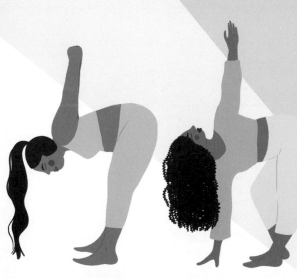

**FORWARD BEND
SHOULDER OPENER**

**FORWARD BEND
WITH TWIST**

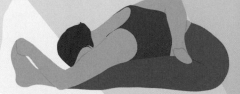

**HALF BOUND
FORWARD BEND**

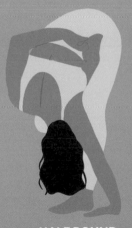

HALF BOUND FORWARD BEND

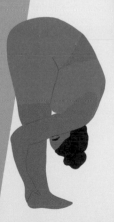

STANDING FORWARD BEND

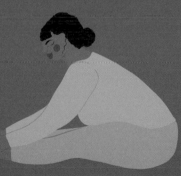

SEATED FORWARD BEND

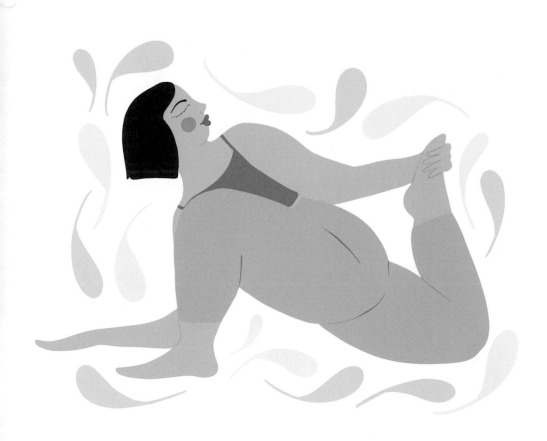

CROOKED MONKEY ON FOREARM

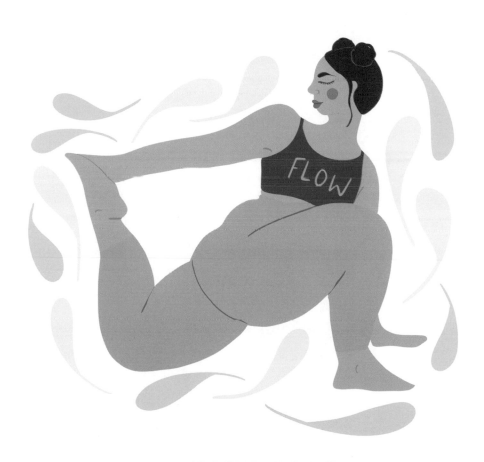

CROOKED MONKEY

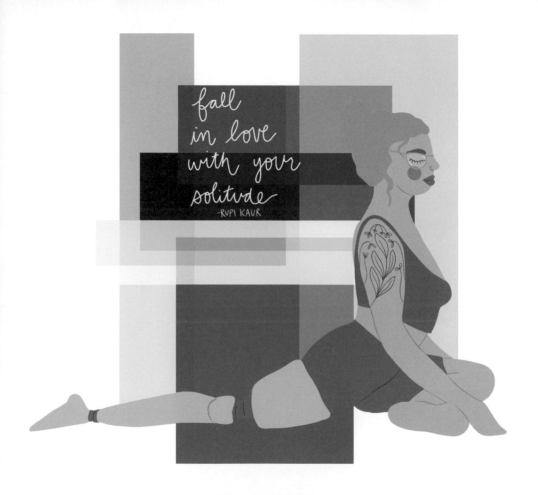

HALF PIGEON
Ardha Kapotāsana

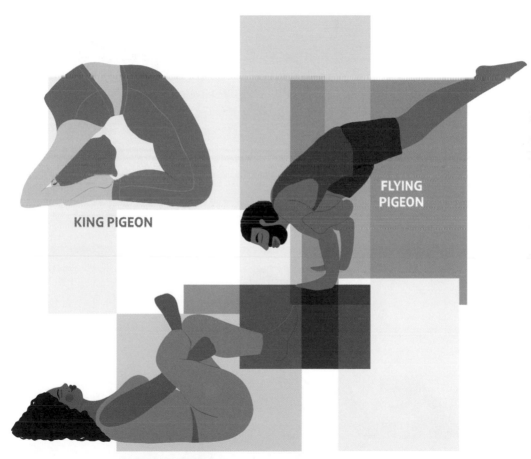

KING PIGEON

FLYING PIGEON

SUPINE PIGEON

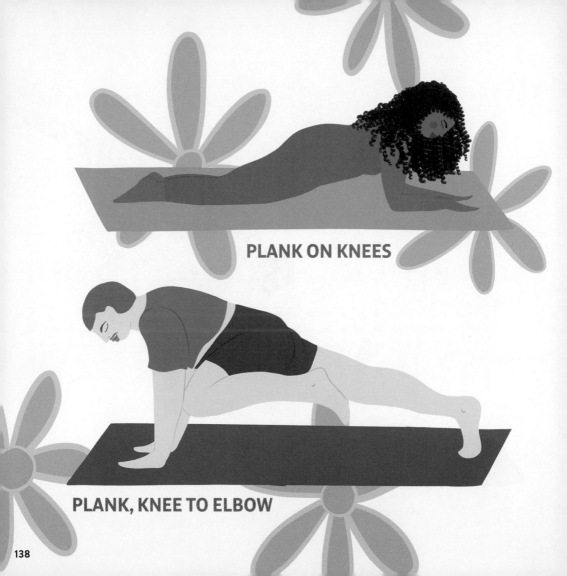

PLANK ON KNEES

PLANK, KNEE TO ELBOW

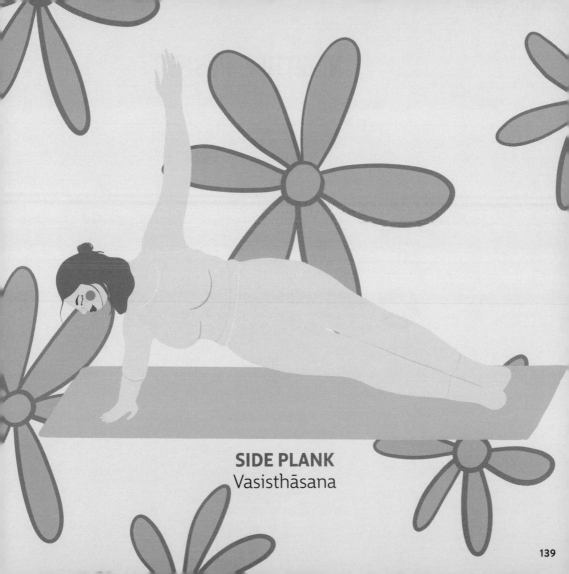

SIDE PLANK
Vasisthāsana

NIGHTTIME POSES

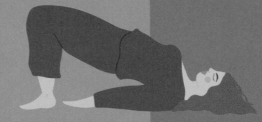

BRIDGE

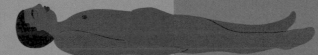

CORPSE

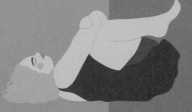

KNEE TO CHEST

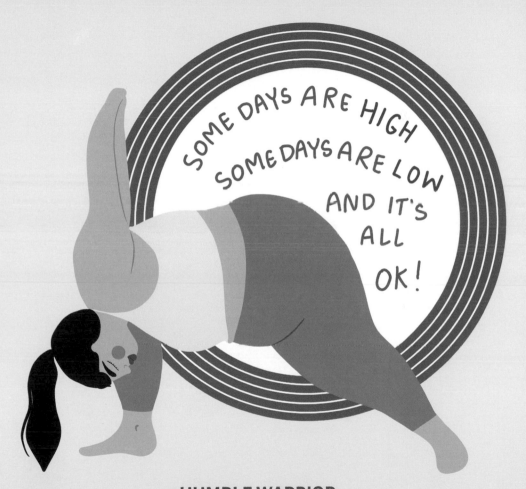

HUMBLE WARRIOR
Baddha Vīrabhadrāsana

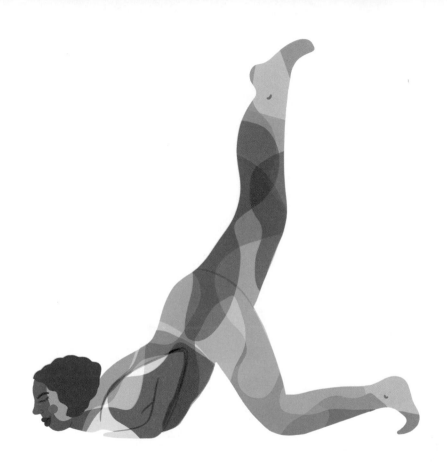

ONE-LEGGED CHIN STAND
Gaṇḍa Bheruṇḍāsana

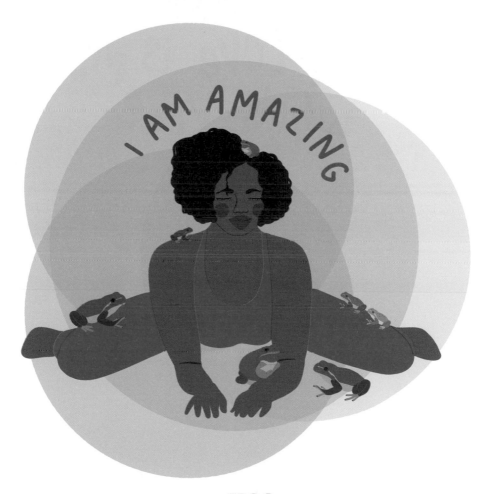

FROG
Mandukāsāna

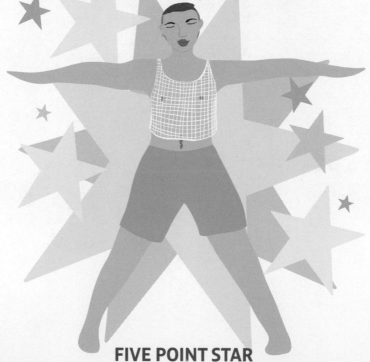

Self-love is my whole vibe

FIVE POINT STAR
Utthita Tādāsana

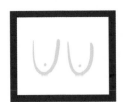

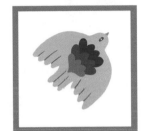

I AM GROWING INTO MYSELF

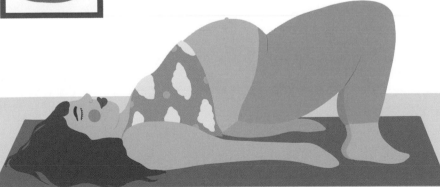

BRIDGE
Setu Bandha Sarvāṅgāsana

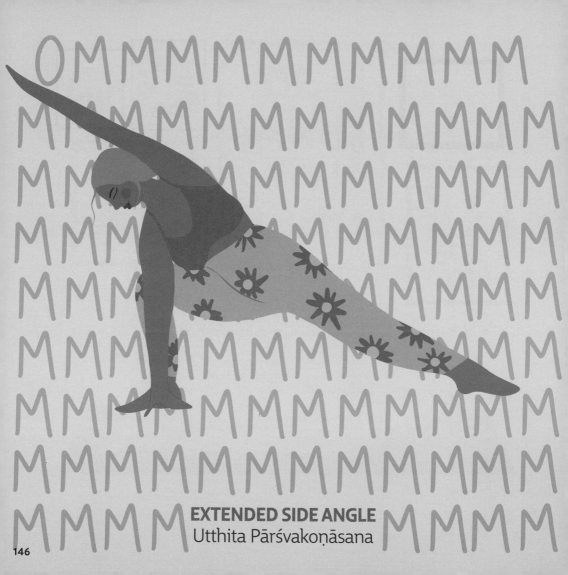

EXTENDED SIDE ANGLE
Utthita Pārśvakoṇāsana

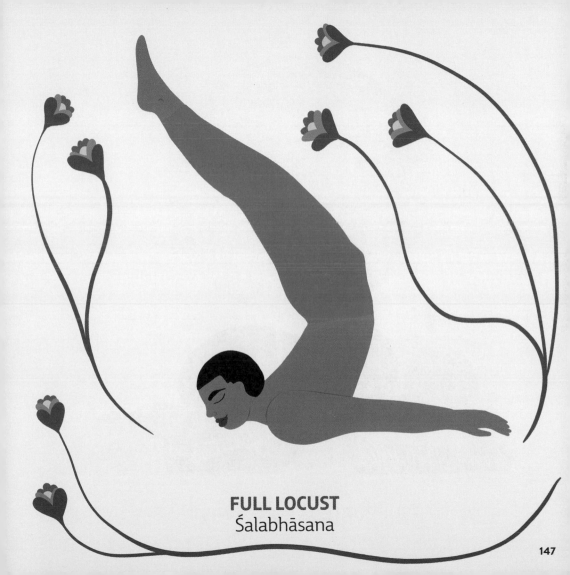

FULL LOCUST
Śalabhāsana

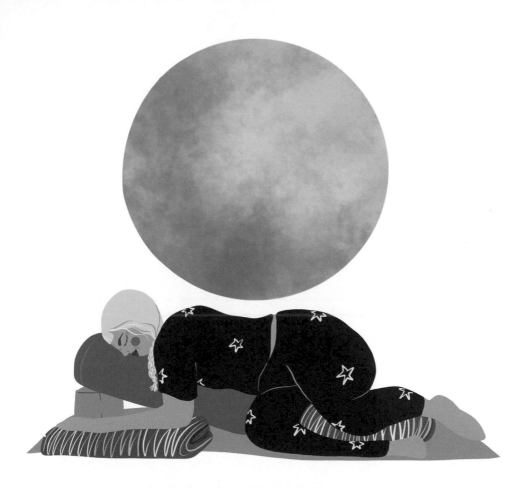

SUPPORTED PRONE TWIST

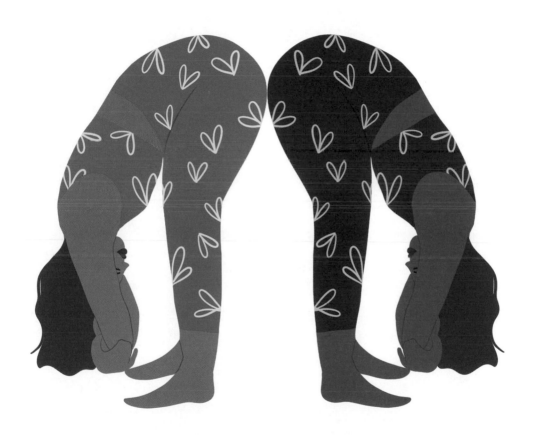

RAGDOLL
Uttānāsana

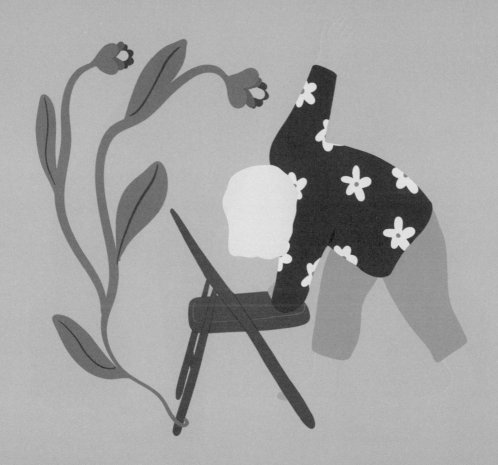

FORWARD BEND WITH EXTENDED ARM
Parivrtta Prasārita Pādottānāsana

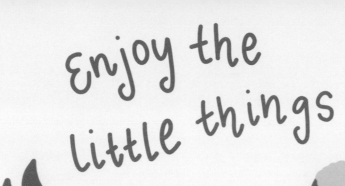

Enjoy the little things

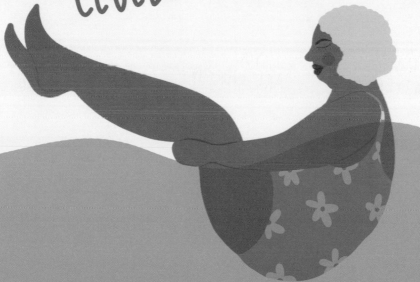

BOAT
Nāvāsana

YOU
MATTER

YOU
ARE WORTHY

YOU ARE
DESERVING

YOU ARE
NEEDED

YOU ARE
VALUED

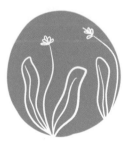

YOU ARE
GOOD

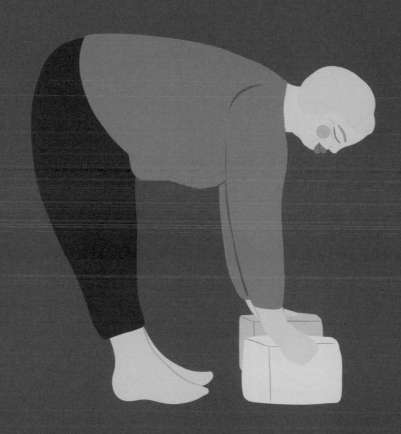

FORWARD BEND

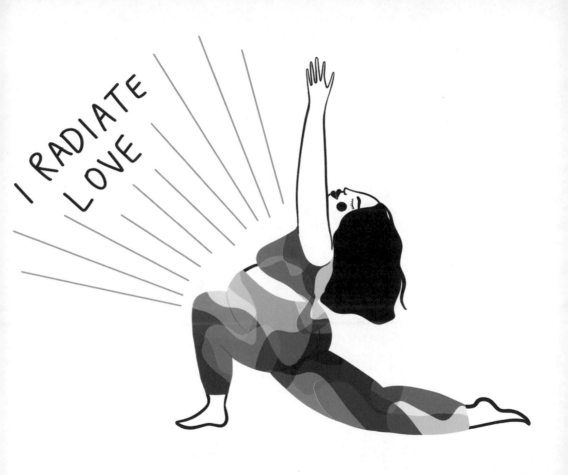

I RADIATE LOVE

LOW LUNGE
Añjaneyāsana

154

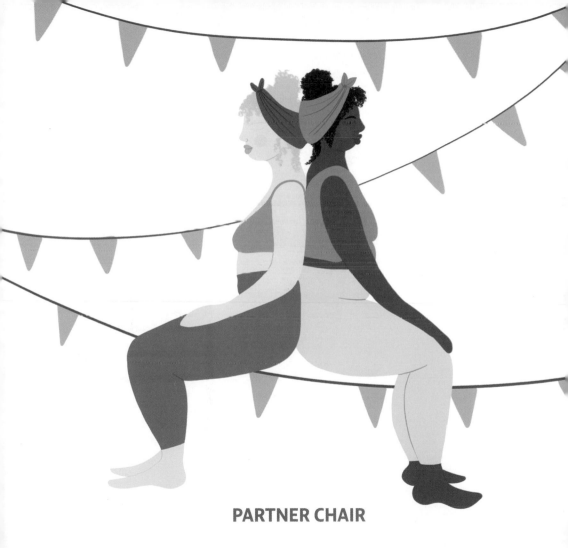

PARTNER CHAIR

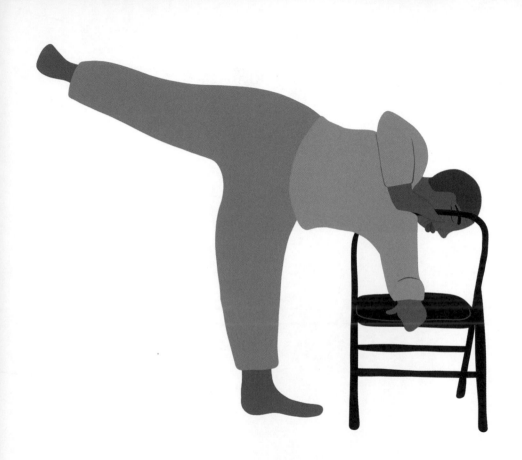

HALF MOON
Ardha Chandrāsana

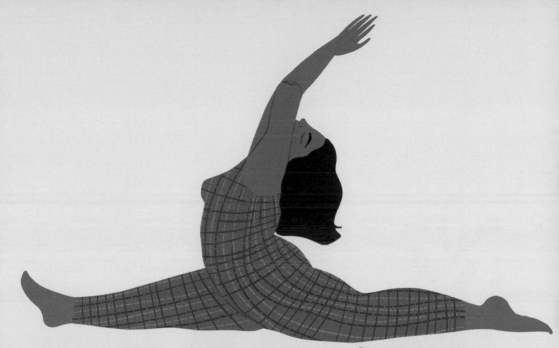

DARE TO BELIEVE IN YOURSELF

FRONT SPLIT
Hanumānāsana

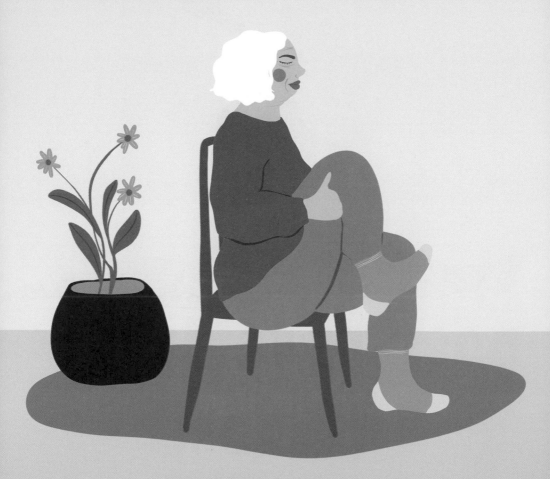

HIP FLEXOR STRETCH

I DECIDE WHO I BECOME

DOLPHIN
Ardha Pīñca Mayūrāsana

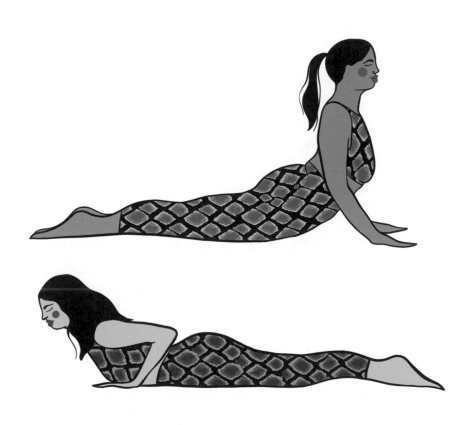

COBRA & BABY COBRA
Bhujaṅgāsana

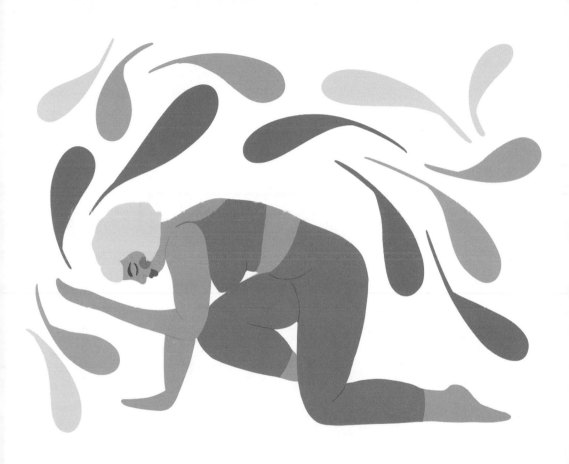

ELBOW TO KNEE
Parivrtta Vrksasana

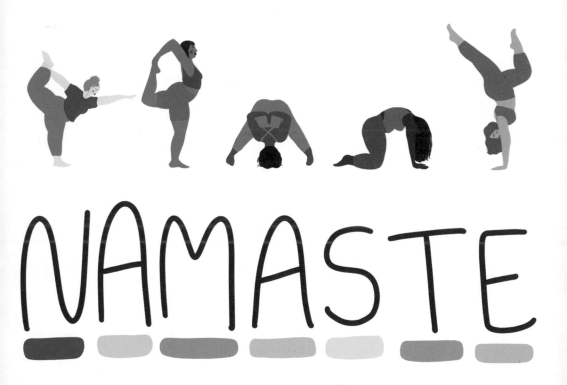

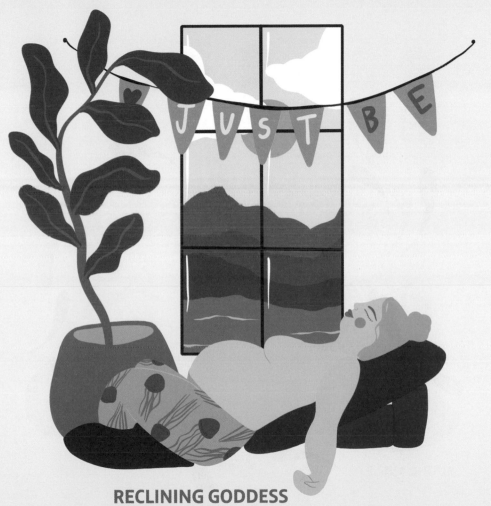

RECLINING GODDESS
Supta Baddha Koṇāsana

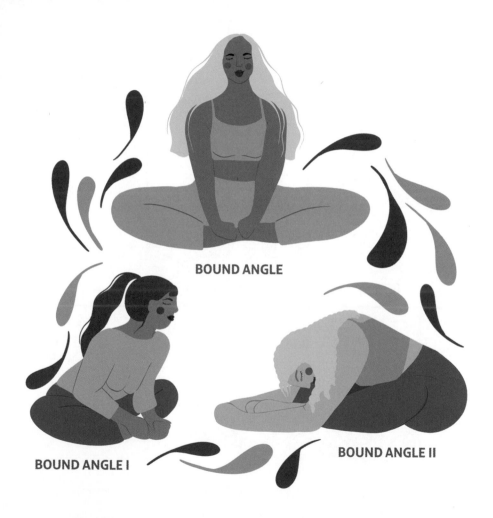

BOUND ANGLE

BOUND ANGLE I

BOUND ANGLE II

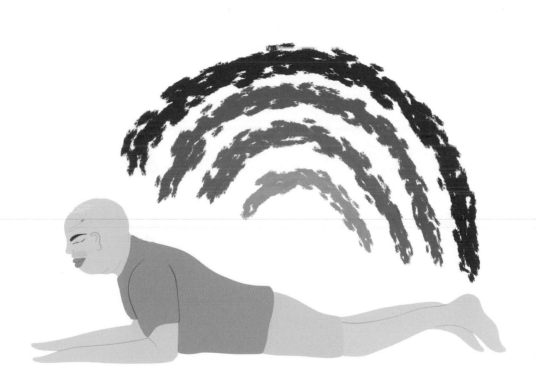

SPHINX
Sālamba Bhujangāsana

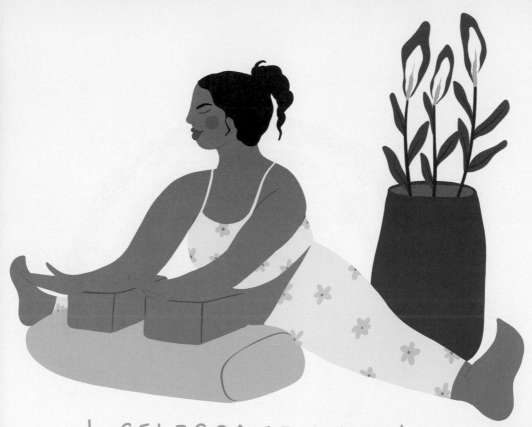

I CELEBRATE WHO I AM

WIDE-LEGGED FORWARD FOLD
Prasārita Pādottānāsana

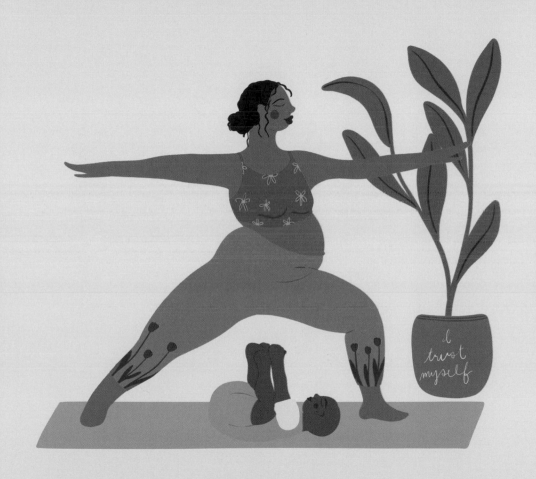

WARRIOR II
Vīrabhadrāsana II

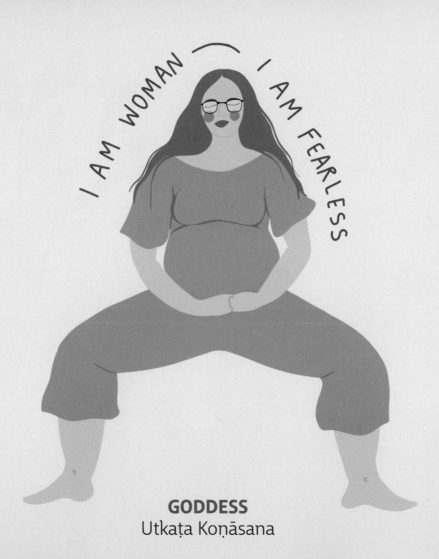

GODDESS
Utkaṭa Koṇāsana

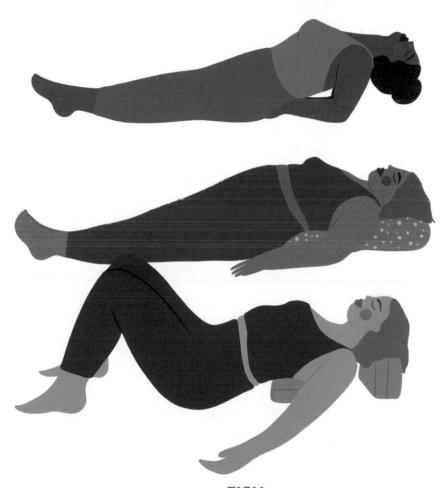

FISH
Matsyāsana

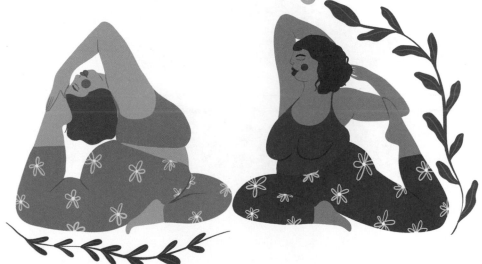

ONE-LEGGED KING PIGEON
Eka Pāda Rajakapotāsana

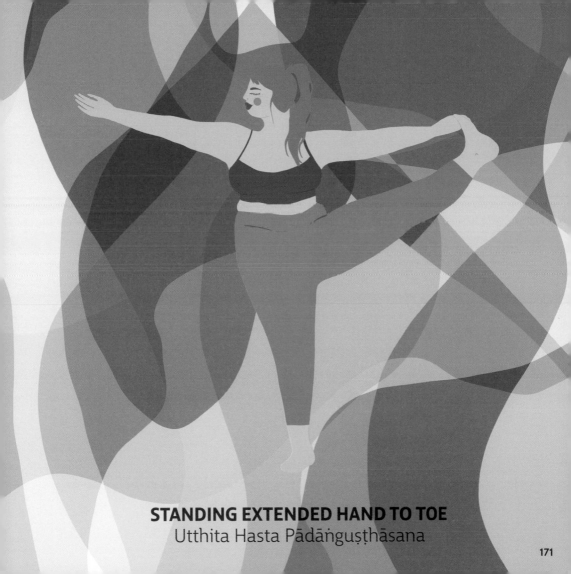

STANDING EXTENDED HAND TO TOE
Utthita Hasta Pādāṅguṣṭhāsana

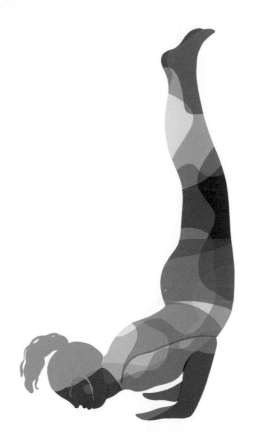
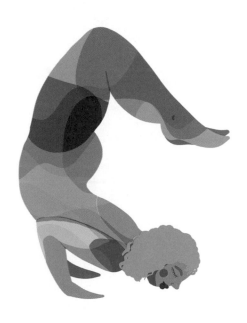

CHIN STAND
Gaṇḍa Bheruṇḍāsana

SCORPION CHIN STAND

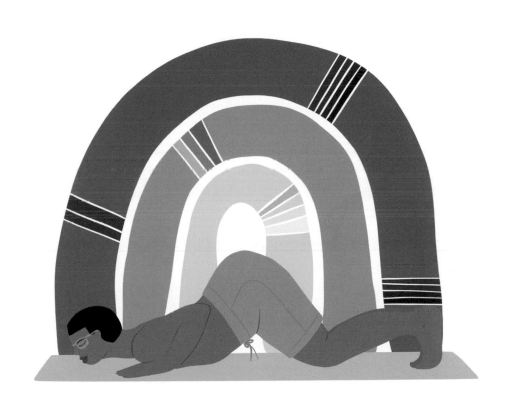

EIGHT POINT
Aṣṭāṅgāsana

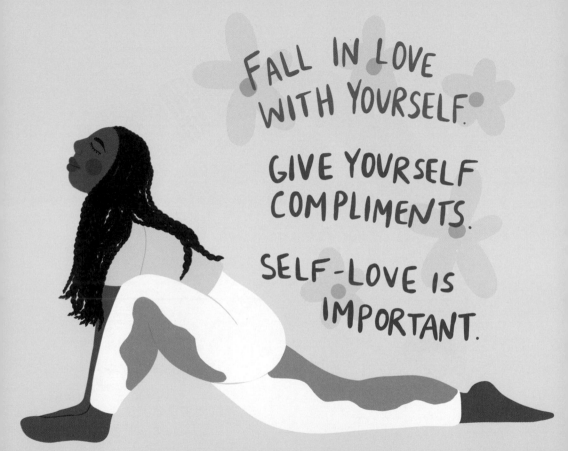

LIZARD ON THE KNEE
Utthan Pristhāsana

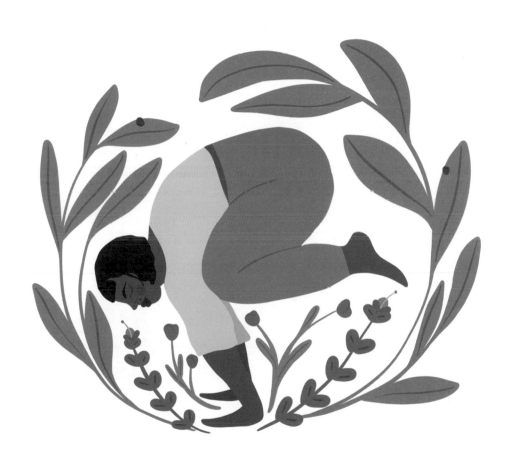

CRANE
Bakāsana

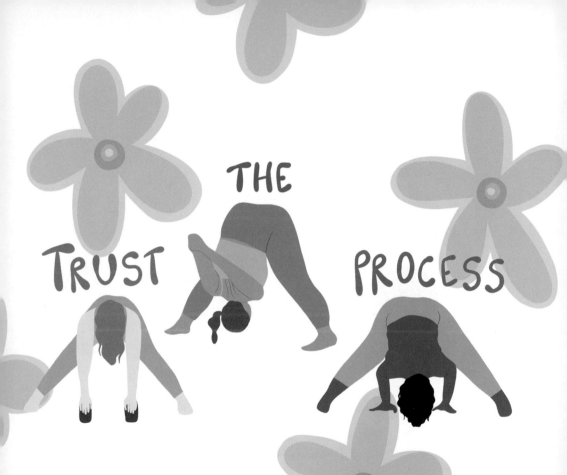

WIDE-LEGGED FORWARD BEND
Prasārita Pādottānāsana I

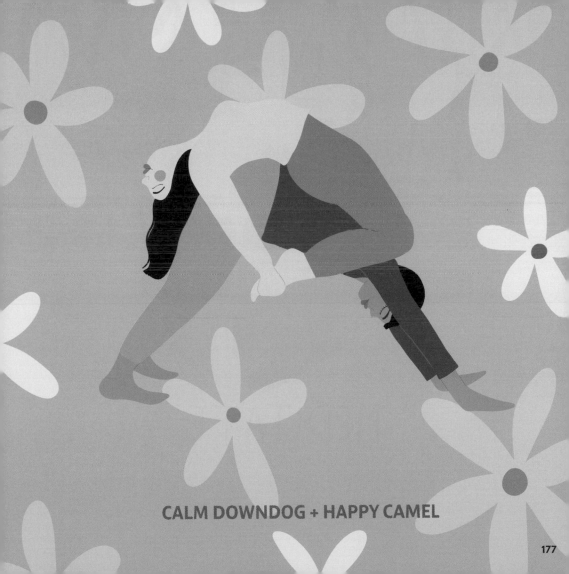

CALM DOWNDOG + HAPPY CAMEL

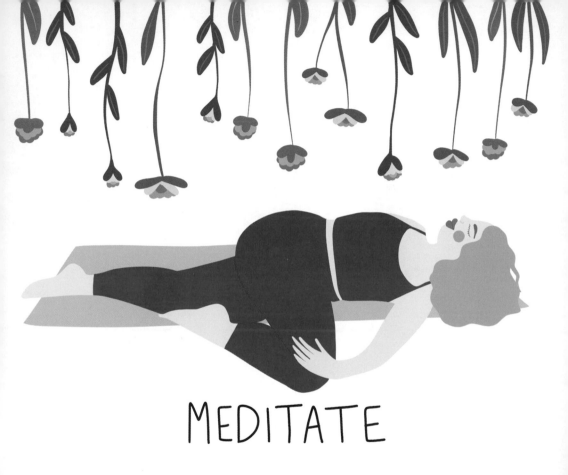

MEDITATE

SUPINE SPINAL TWIST
Supta Matsyendrāsana

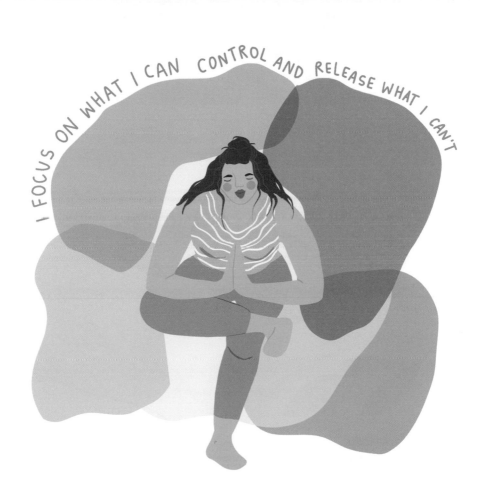

I FOCUS ON WHAT I CAN CONTROL AND RELEASE WHAT I CAN'T

FIGURE FOUR
Eka Pāda Utkaṭāsana

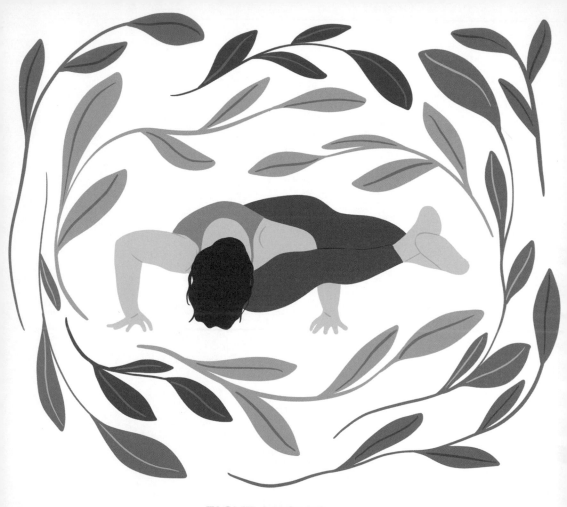

EIGHT ANGLES
Aṣṭāvakrāsana

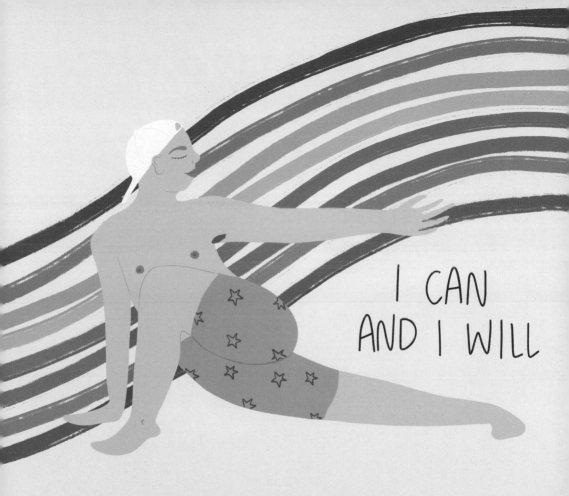

I CAN
AND I WILL

HORIZON LUNGE

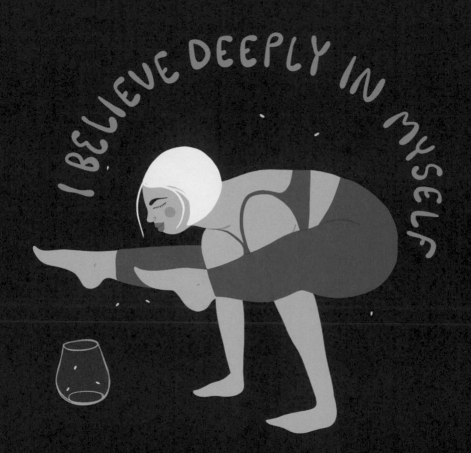

I BELIEVE DEEPLY IN MYSELF

FIREFLY
Tittibhāsana

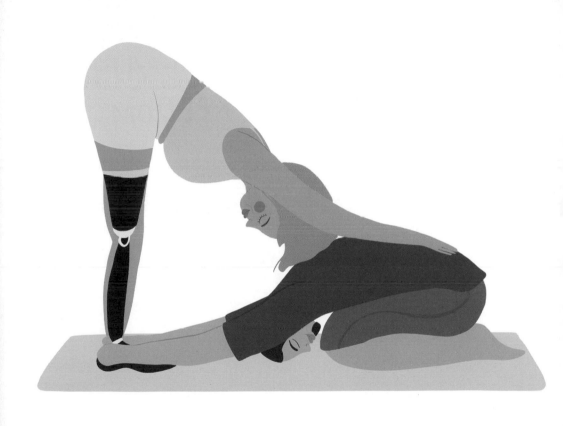

FORWARD BEND + CHILD'S POSE

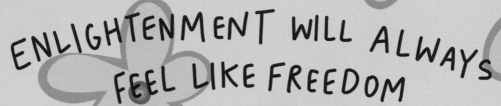

ENLIGHTENMENT WILL ALWAYS FEEL LIKE FREEDOM

—BUDDHA

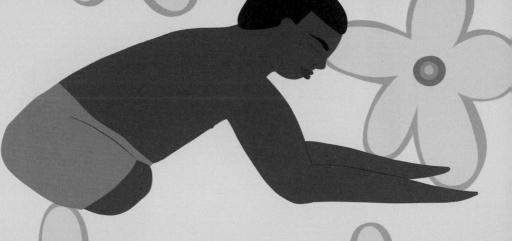

**WIDE-ANGLE
SEATED FORWARD BEND**

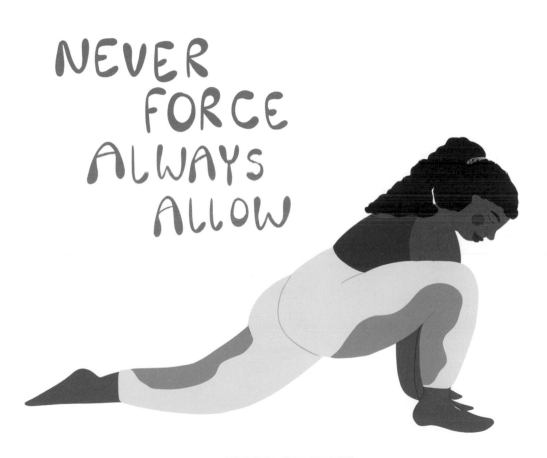

NEVER
FORCE
ALWAYS
ALLOW

LIZARD ON KNEE
Utthan Pristhāsana

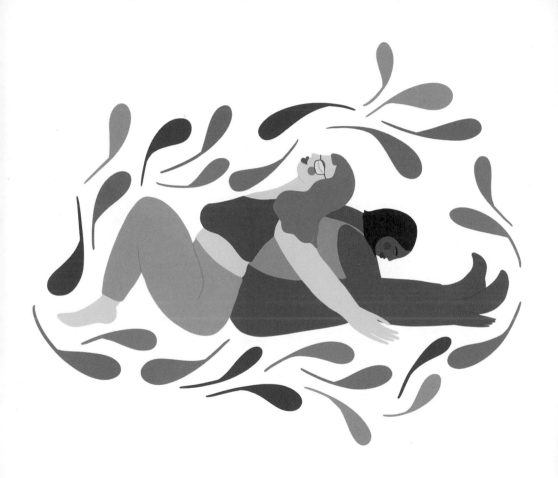

FORWARD FOLD + BACK BEND

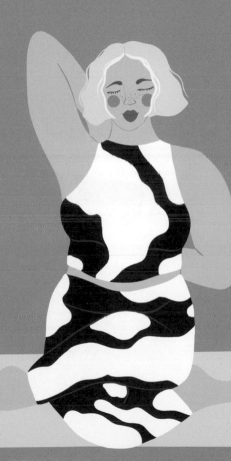

SELF-
LOVE
IS THE
BEST
LOVE

COW FACE
Gomukhāsana

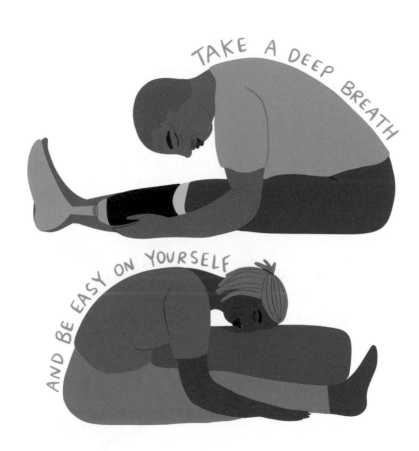

CATERPILLAR
Paschimottānāsana

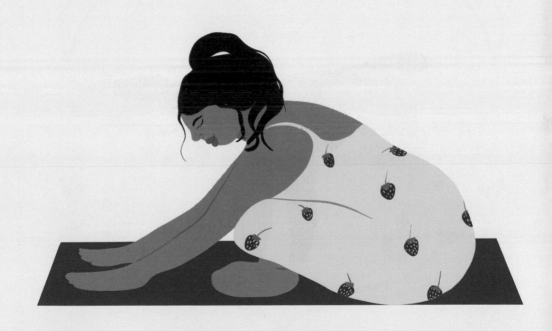

FORWARD BEND FIRE LOG
Agnistambhāsana

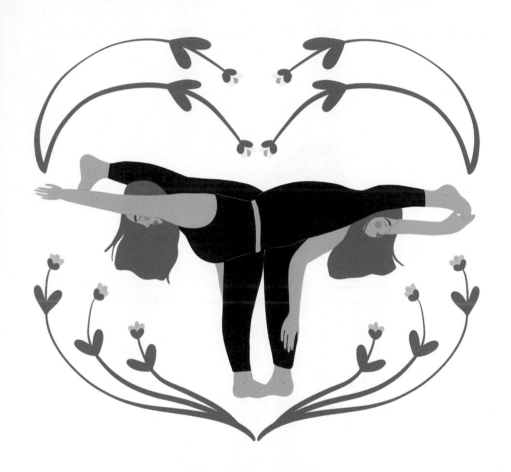

INTERTWINED TWINS

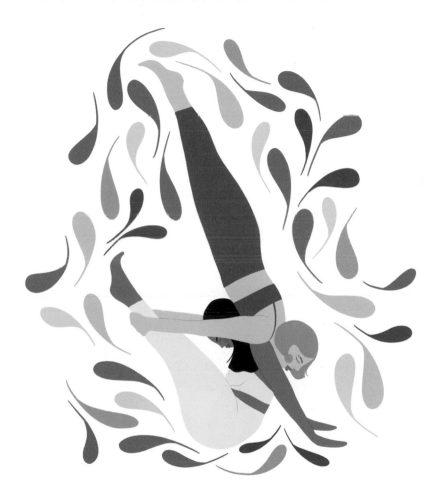

BACK SLIDE

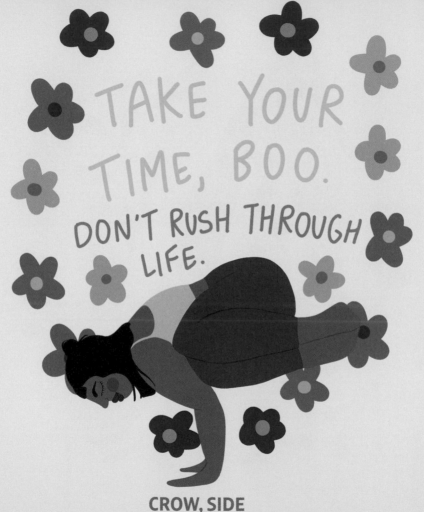

CROW, SIDE
Pārśva Bakāsana

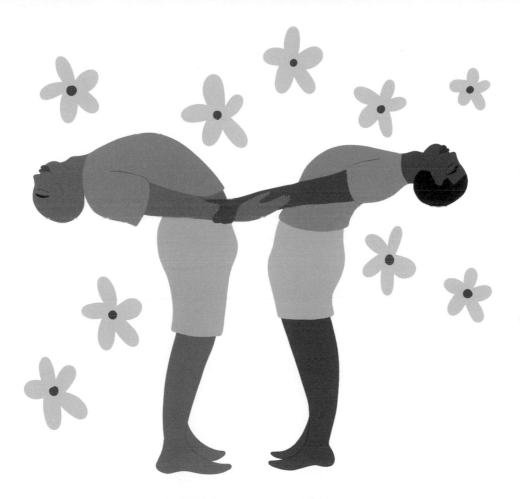

PARTNER BACKBEND

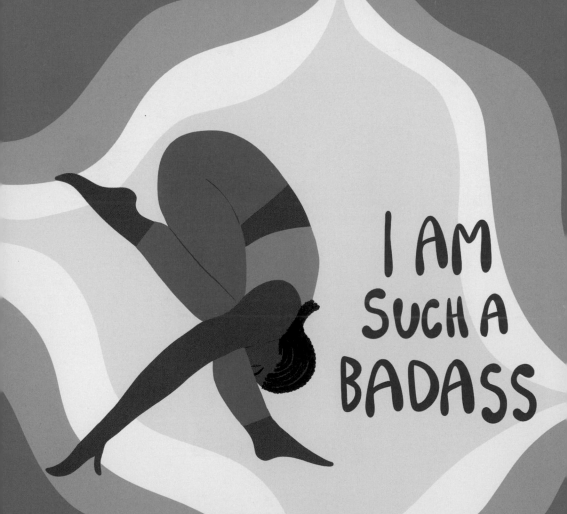

I AM SUCH A BADASS

HUMBLE FLAMINGO

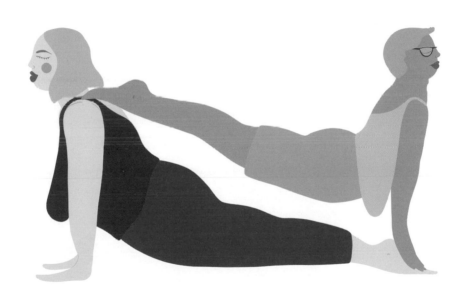

PARTNERED PLANKS

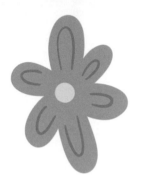

I AM
GRATEFUL

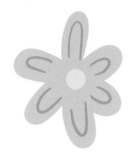

I CAN DO
HARD THINGS

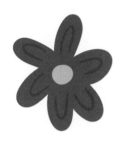

I RESPECT
MYSELF

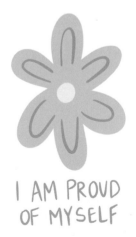

I AM PROUD
OF MYSELF

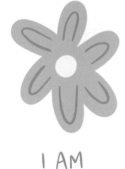

I AM
WHOLE

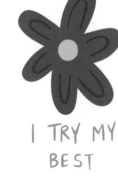

I TRY MY
BEST

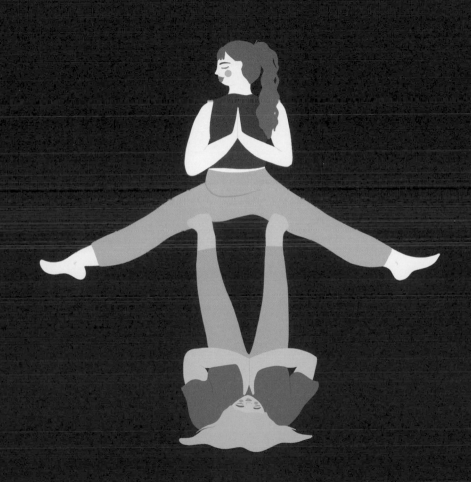

RISING GODDESS

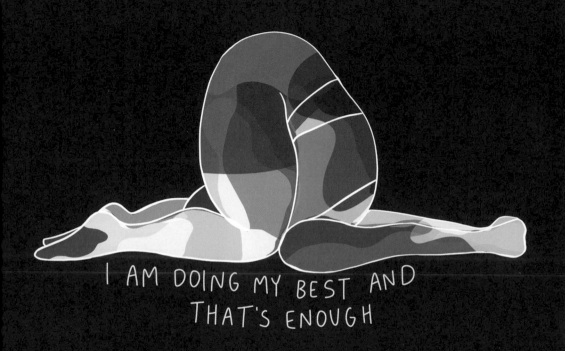

I AM DOING MY BEST AND THAT'S ENOUGH

EAR PRESSURE POSE
Karṇapīḍāsana

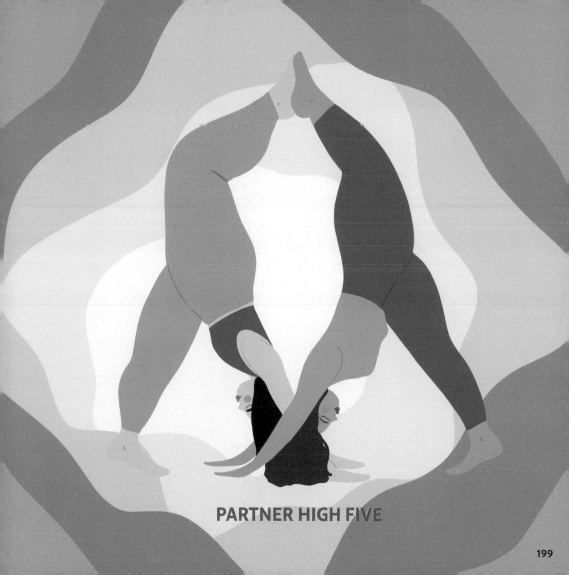

PARTNER HIGH FIVE

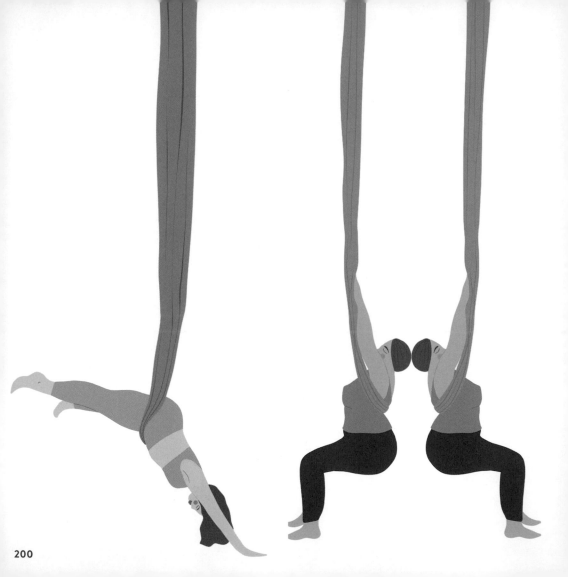

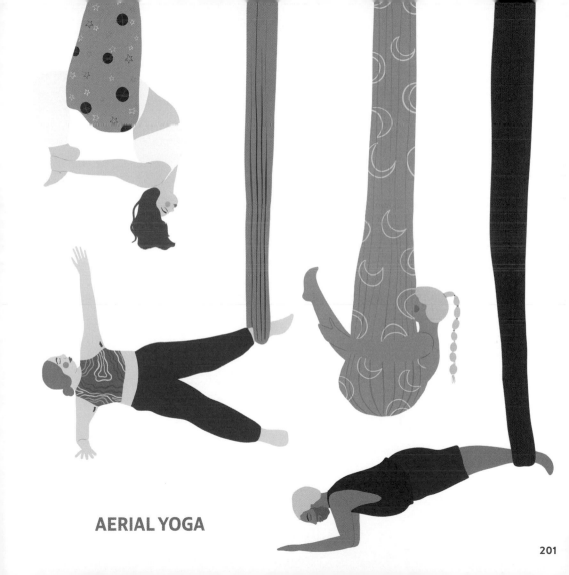

AERIAL YOGA

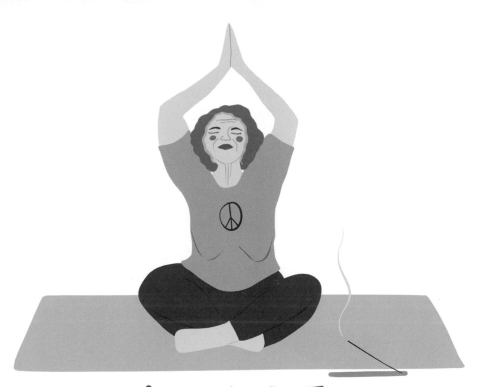

I AM KIND TO MYSELF

LOTUS
Padmāsana

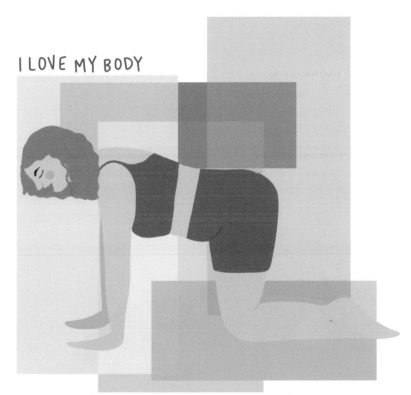

I LOVE MY BODY

AND ALL THAT IT DOES FOR ME

TABLE
Cakravākāsana

THE BEST INVESTMENT TO MAKE IS IN YOURSELF

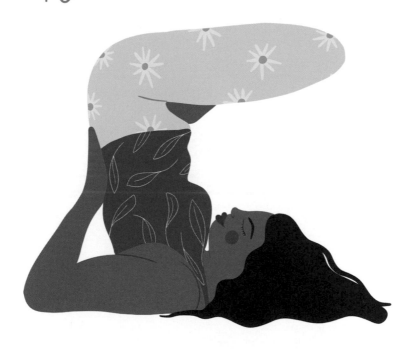

SHOULDER STAND, LOTUS LEGS
Ūrdhva Padmāsana

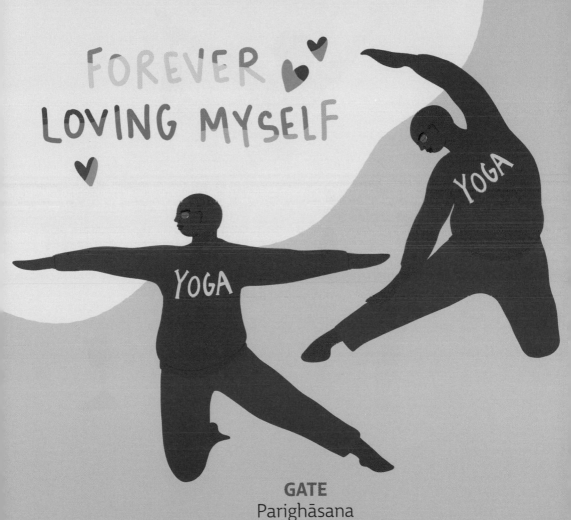

GATE
Parighāsana

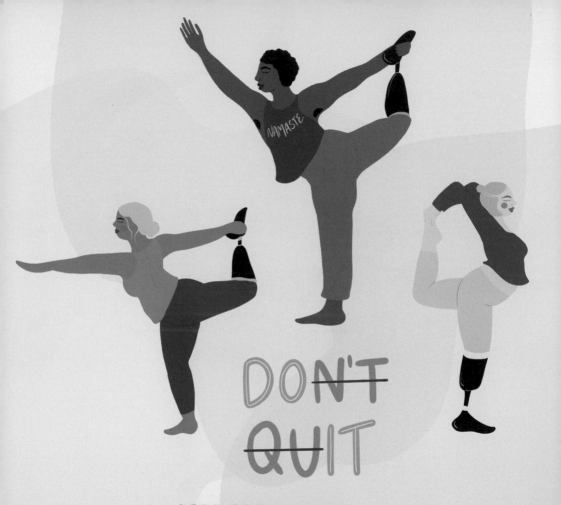

LORD OF THE DANCE
Parivṛtta Naṭarājāsana

TRUST THE TIMING OF YOUR LIFE

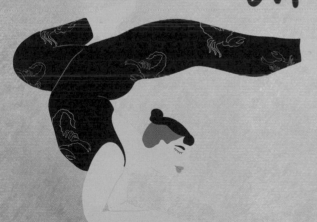
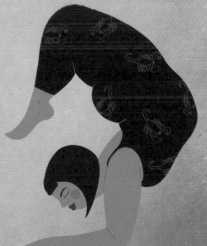

SCORPION
Vrśhikāsana I

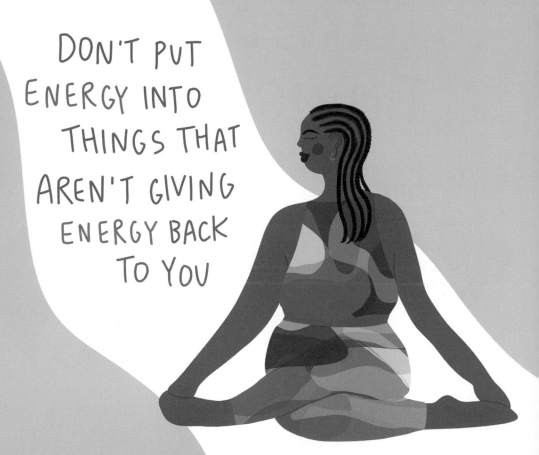

DON'T PUT ENERGY INTO THINGS THAT AREN'T GIVING ENERGY BACK TO YOU

SHOELACE

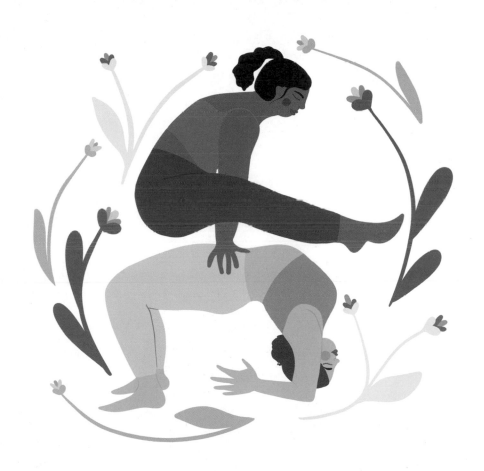

RABBIT HOP

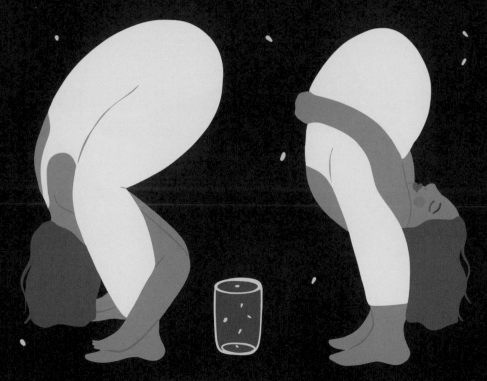

I GLOW FROM WITHIN

STANDING FIREFLY
Utthita Tittibhāsana

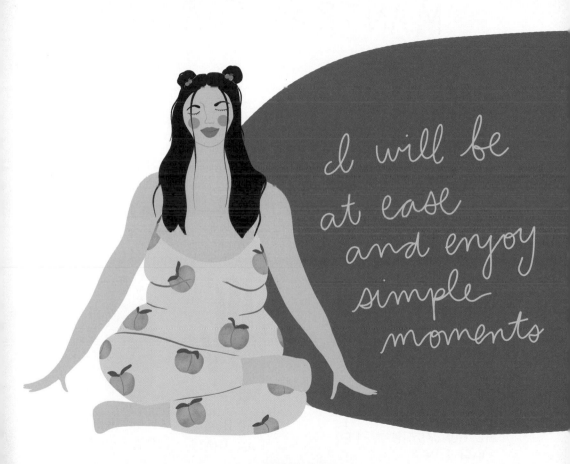

I will be at ease and enjoy simple moments

FIRE LOG
Agnistambhāsana

MANTRAS FOR ME

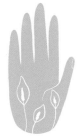

I AM
ENOUGH

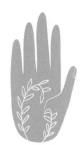

OM

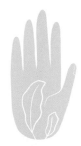

INHALE-
1. 2. 3. 4. 5

EXHALE-
1. 2. 3. 4. 5

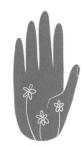

I AM WHERE
MY FEET ARE

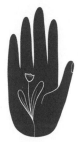

THE LIGHT IN
ME HONORS THE
LIGHT IN
YOU

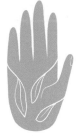

I
LET
GO

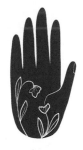

SO HAM
(I AM THAT)

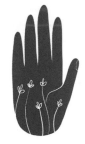

I AM HERE
FOR A PURPOSE

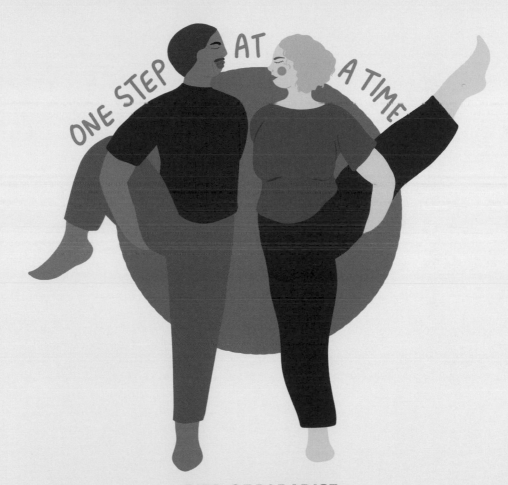

ONE STEP AT A TIME

BIRD OF PARADISE
Svarga Dvijāsana

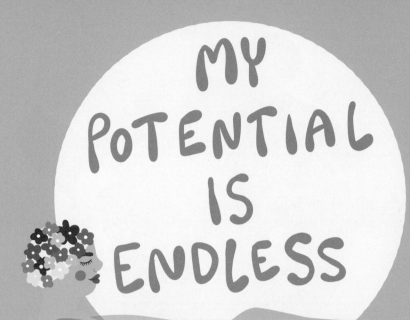

MY POTENTIAL IS ENDLESS

BOAT
Nāvāsana

I AM LOVED — I AM NEEDED

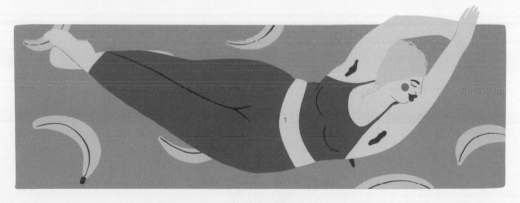

BANANA
Bananāsāna

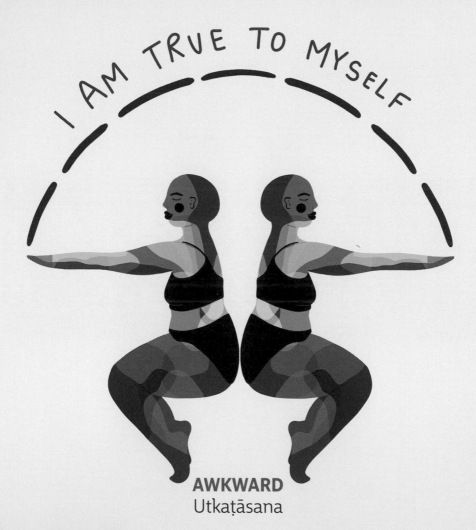

AWKWARD
Utkaṭāsana

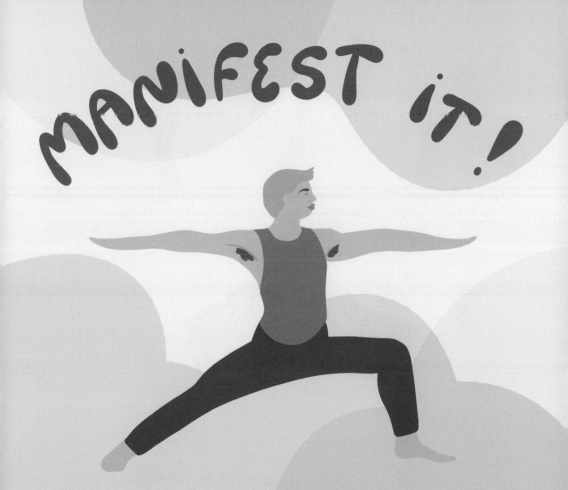

WARRIOR II
Vīrabhadrāsana II

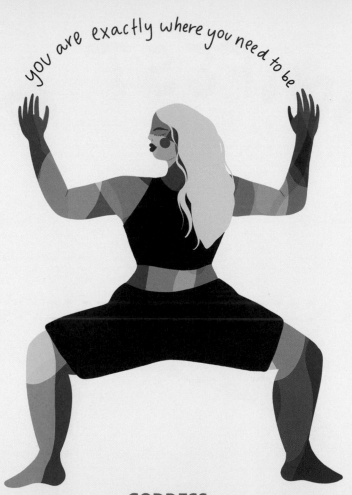

GODDESS
Uṭkaṭa Koṇāsana

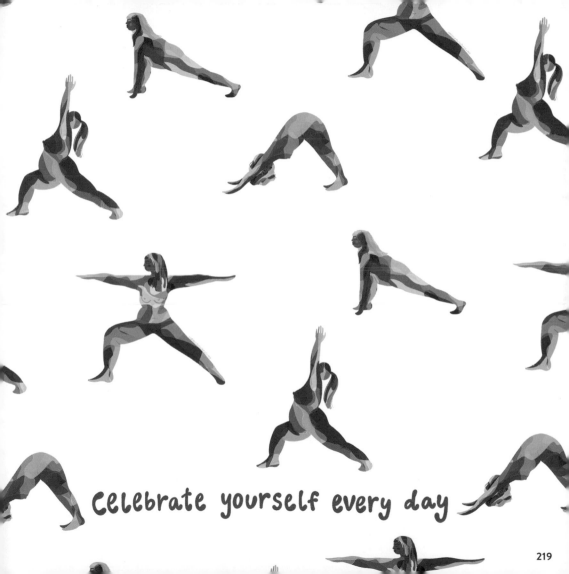

Celebrate yourself every day

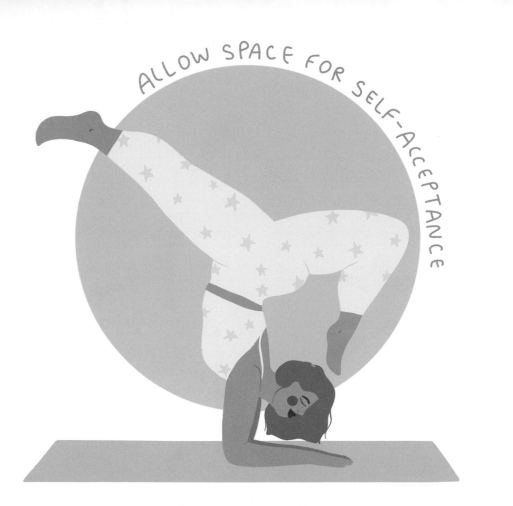

ALLOW SPACE FOR SELF-ACCEPTANCE

FOREARM STAND WITH STAG LEG
Pīñca Mayūrāsana

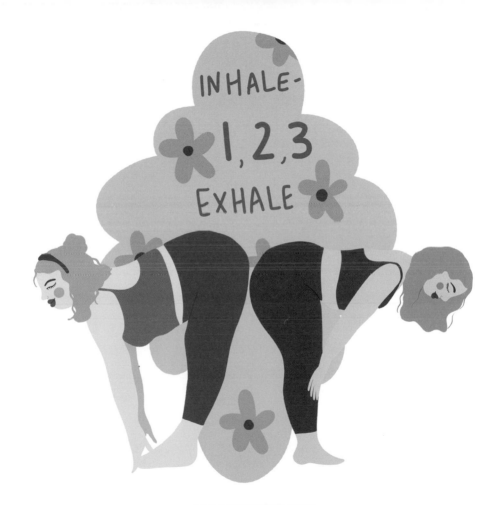

INHALE—
1, 2, 3
EXHALE

HALFWAY LIFT
Ardha Uttanāsana

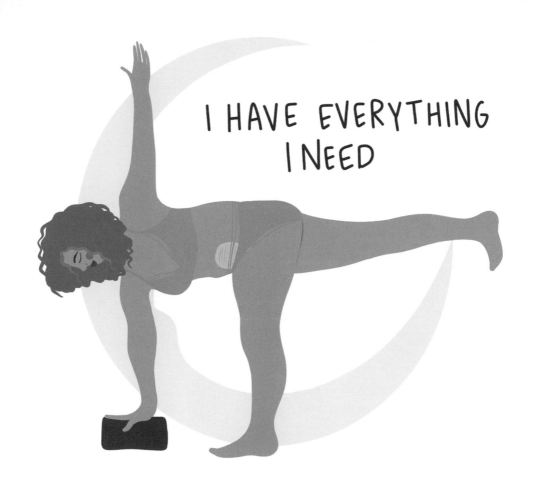

I HAVE EVERYTHING I NEED

HALF MOON
Ardha Chandrāsana

222

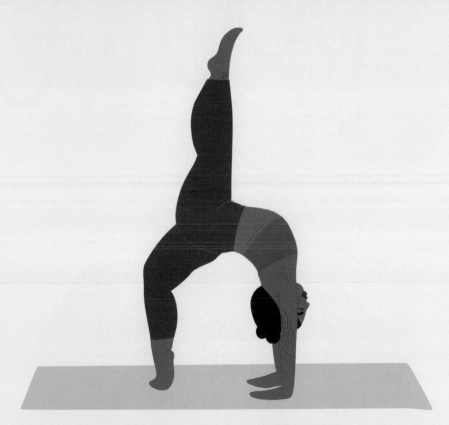

I AM MY HEALING

ONE-LEGGED WHEEL
Eka Pāda Ūrdhva Dhanurāsana

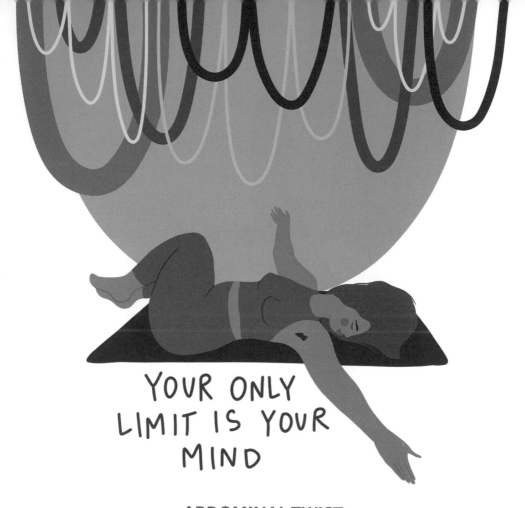

ABDOMINAL TWIST
Jathara Parivartanasana

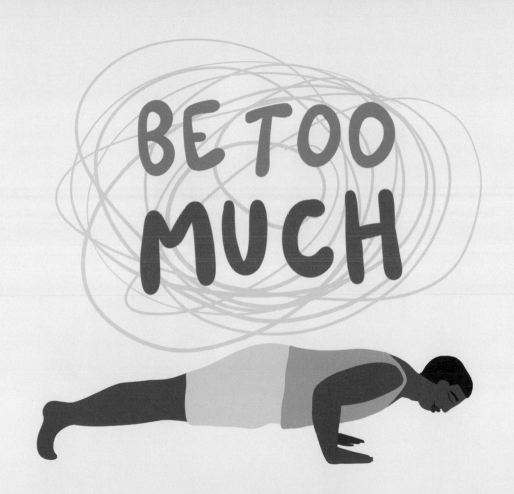

FOUR-LIMBED STAFF
Caturaṅga Daṇḍāsana

I CHOOSE ME

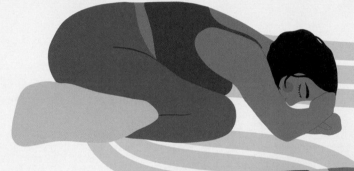

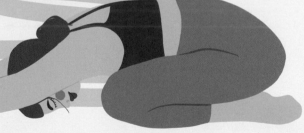

CHILD'S POSE
Bālāsana

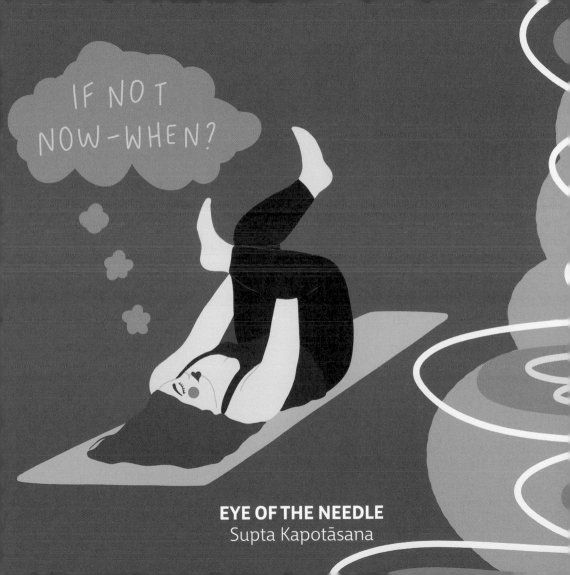

EYE OF THE NEEDLE
Supta Kapotāsana

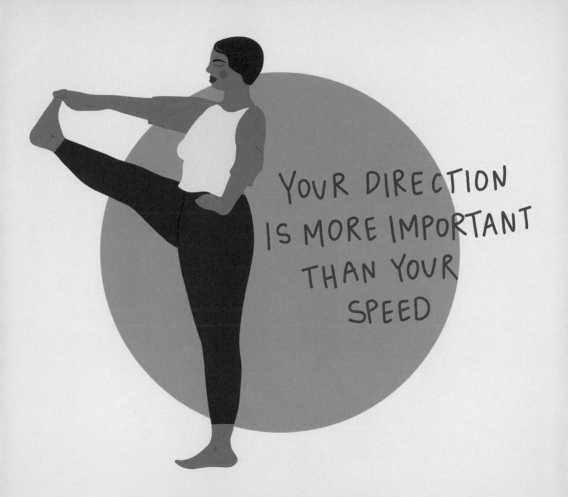

YOUR DIRECTION IS MORE IMPORTANT THAN YOUR SPEED

EXTENDED HAND TO TOE
Utthita Hasta Pādāngusthāsana

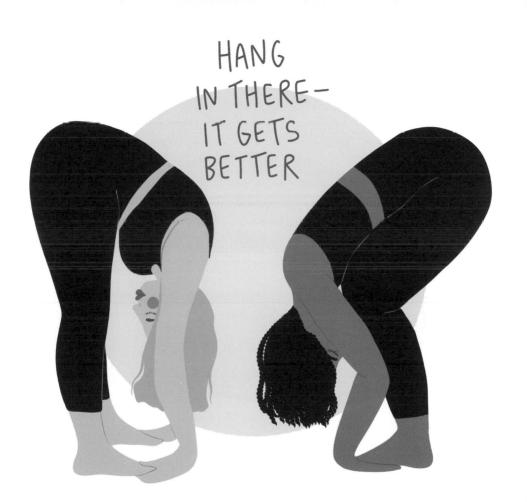

GORILLA
Pādahastāsana

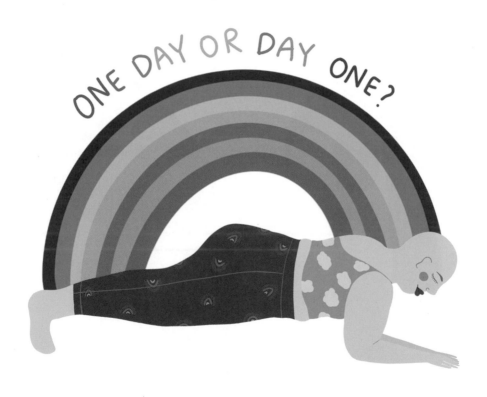

FOREARM PLANK
Phalakasana II

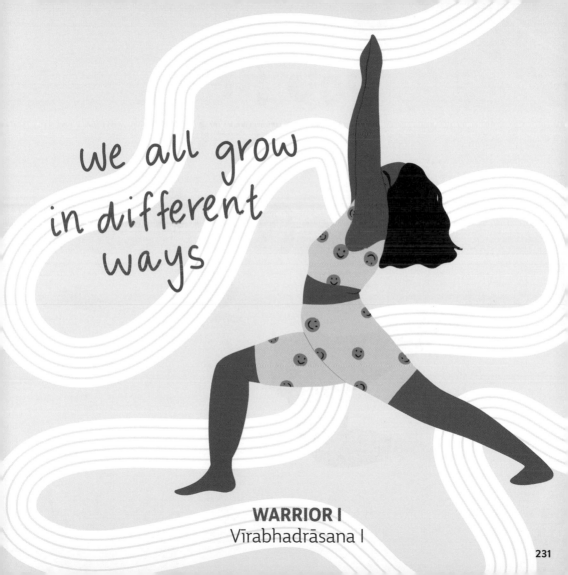

we all grow
in different
ways

WARRIOR I
Vīrabhadrāsana I

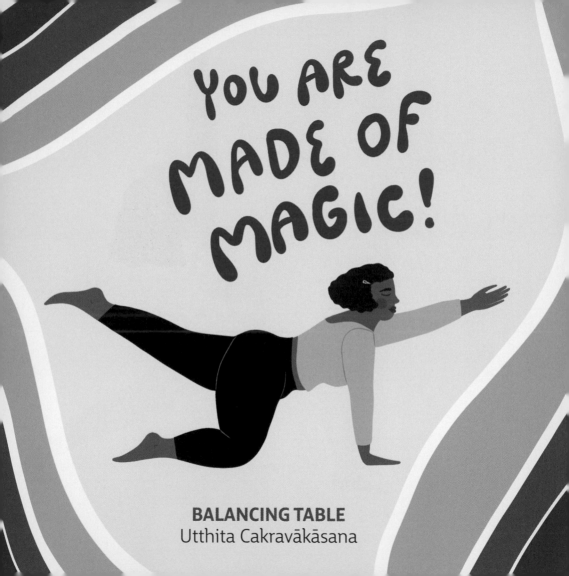

BALANCING TABLE
Utthita Cakravākāsana

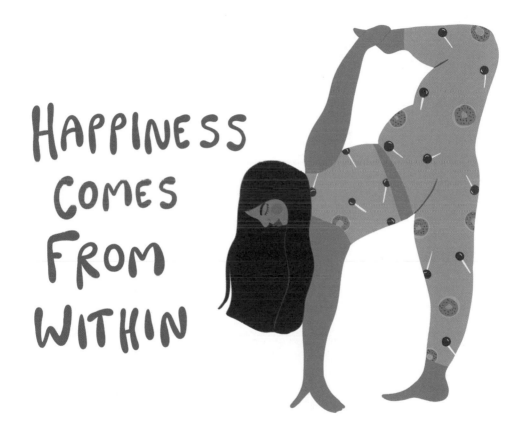

HAPPINESS COMES FROM WITHIN

SUGARCANE
Ardha Candra Cāpāsana

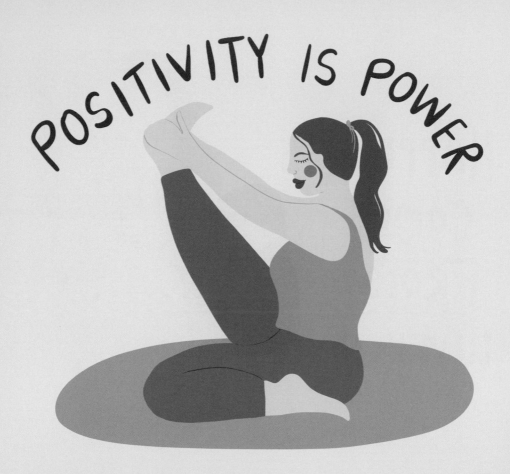

HERON
Krauñcāsana

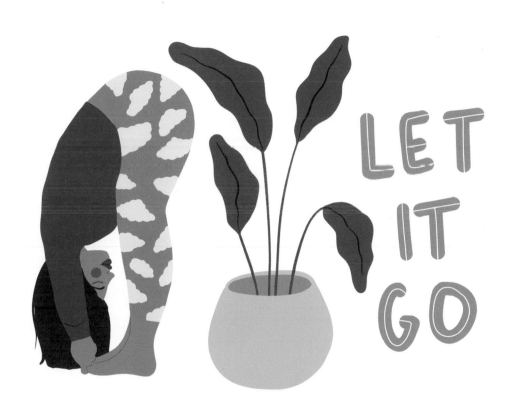

BIG TOE POSE
Pādāṅguṣṭhāsana

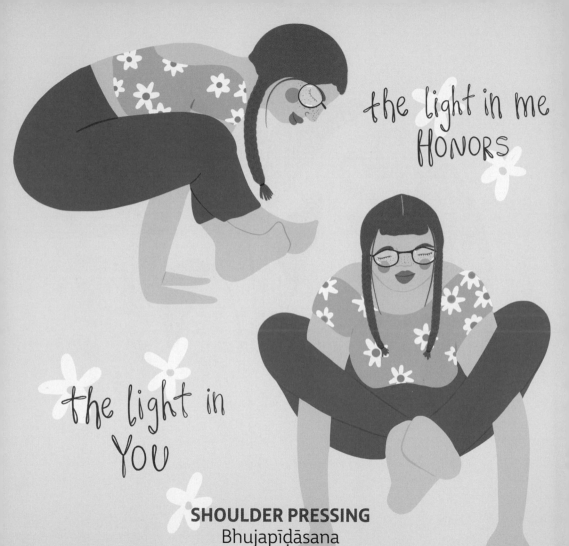

the light in me HONORS

the light in YOU

SHOULDER PRESSING
Bhujapīḍāsana

I AM MAKING A GREAT LIFE

WARRIOR III
Vīrabhadrāsana III

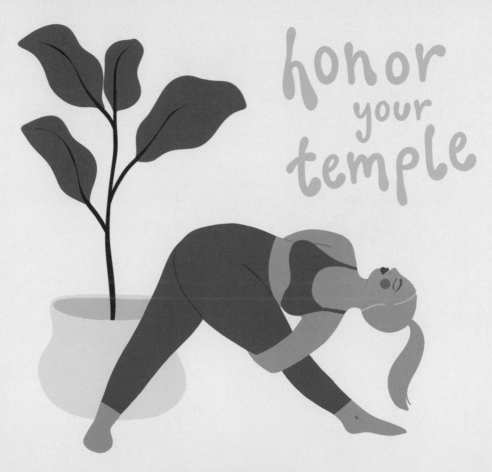

honor your temple

BOUND TRIANGLE
Baddha Trikoṇāsana

I AM THE AUTHOR OF MY OWN STORY

UPWARD-FACING DOG
Ūrdhva Mukha Śvānāsana

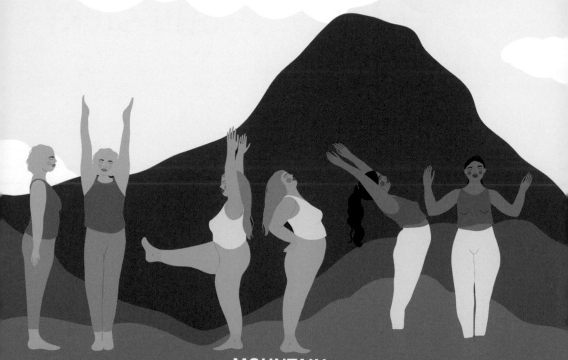

MOUNTAIN
Tāḍāsana

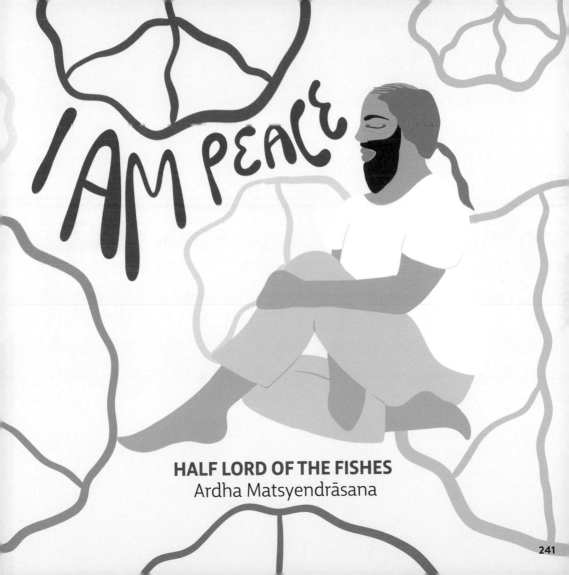

HALF LORD OF THE FISHES
Ardha Matsyendrāsana

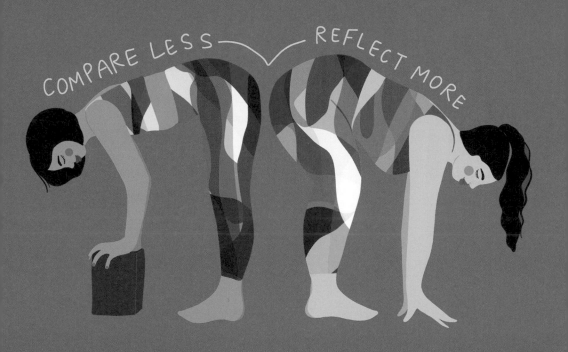

COMPARE LESS — REFLECT MORE

FORWARD
Uttānāsana

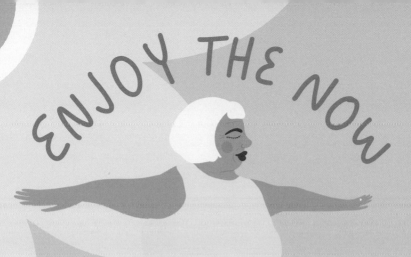

ENJOY THE NOW

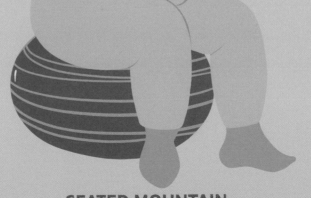

SEATED MOUNTAIN
Parvatasana

ACKNOWLEDGMENTS

I would like to thank my parents who have always believed in me and been incredibly proud of all my accomplishments. Mom, thank you for passing down your gift of creativity and imagination, and Dad, thank you for giving me a solid foundation to grow from. My sister, Adeline, who is both my biggest fan but also always there to challenge me and make me dig deeper. Charlotte, Jackson, and Henry, who always told me everything I drew was beautiful. Emily, who I have always looked up to and whose goddess vibrations I will always be in awe of. Megan, who encouraged me to follow my dreams of illustrating. All of my beautiful friends: Amelia, Tayler, Bianca, AJ, Asha, Laura, Damas, Aurelia, and Alexa, who have been the best cheerleaders and always believed in me.

At Workman, thank you to Anna for finding my work, Mary Ellen for giving me this opportunity, Kim for shepherding, Lisa for designing, and Rebecca and Claire for marketing and publicity. Thank you to all my friends and family who have been both inspiration and encouragement. I wouldn't have been able to create this book without all of your love and support. Thank you.

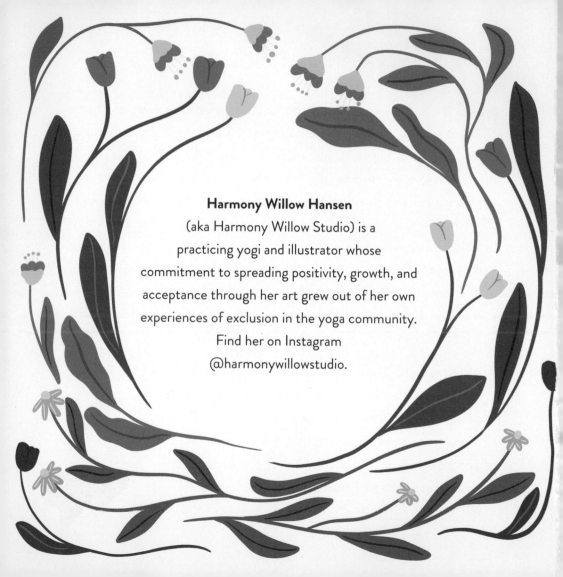

Harmony Willow Hansen
(aka Harmony Willow Studio) is a
practicing yogi and illustrator whose
commitment to spreading positivity, growth, and
acceptance through her art grew out of her own
experiences of exclusion in the yoga community.
Find her on Instagram
@harmonywillowstudio.